Compliance Issues in Ophthalmology

EDITED BY ALAN REIDER, MPH, JD

Arent, Fox, Kintner, Plotkin, & Kahn, PLLC
Washington, DC

SLACK
INCORPORATED

An innovative information, education, and management company
6900 Grove Road • Thorofare, NJ 08086

The procedures and practices described in this book should be implemented in a manner consistent with the professional standards set for the circumstances that apply in each specific situation. Every effort has been made to confirm the accuracy of the information presented and to correctly relate generally accepted practices. The author, editor, and publisher cannot accept responsibility for errors or exclusions or for the outcome of the application of the material presented herein. There is no expressed or implied warranty of this book or information imparted by it.

Printed in the United States of America.

Library of Congress Cataloging-in-Publication Data
Compliance issues in ophthalmology / edited by Alan Reider.
    p. ; cm.
Includes bibliographical references and index.
  ISBN 1-55642-613-5 (pbk. : alk. paper)
  1. Ophthalmology--Practice.
  [DNLM: 1. Insurance Claim Reporting--legislation &
jurisprudence--United States. 2. Ophthalmology--standards--United
States. 3. Guideline Adherence--United States. 4. Insurance, Health,
Reimbursement--legislation & jurisprudence--United States. 5.
Medicare--legislation & jurisprudence. W 21 C7375 2002] I. Reider,
Alan E.
  RE72 .C66 2002
  617.7'0068--dc21
                                                                    2002007744

Published by: SLACK Incorporated
                   6900 Grove Road
                   Thorofare, NJ 08086 USA
                   Telephone: 856-848-1000
                   Fax: 856-853-5991
                   www.slackbooks.com

Contact SLACK Incorporated for more information about other books in this field or about the availability of our books from distributors outside the United States.

Last digit is print number: 10   9   8   7   6   5   4   3   2   1

CONTENTS

About the Editor

Alan E. Reider, MPH, JD joined the law firm of Arent Fox in 1980 after having spent 5 years in the Health Care Financing Administration of the Department of Health & Human Services. During his tenure in the department, Mr. Reider worked in the Office of Program Integrity (now part of the Office of the Inspector General) and the Office of Professional Standards Review Organizations, where he was Chief of the Review Policy Branch.

Mr. Reider's practice is limited to health law. He represents physicians, suppliers, hospitals, laboratories, as well as national health care corporations. This representation focuses on regulatory issues involving federal programs, as well as relationships with third-party payors, counseling in the area of fraud and abuse, principally the federal Anti-Kickback Statute and Stark Self-Referral Law, as well as state restrictions, development of compliance programs, and defending providers and practitioners in False Claims Act, Civil Money Penalty, and suspension and exclusion actions.

Mr. Reider has extensive experience working with ophthalmology practices. He serves as outside counsel to the Society for Excellence in Eyecare as well as the International Society for Refractive Surgery. He is the author of the *Model Compliance Program for Ophthalmologists*, published by the American Society of Ophthalmic Administrators. Mr. Reider serves as the Regulatory and Legislative Section Editor for *Ocular Surgery News*.

Contributing Authors

E. Ann Rose is president of Rose & Associates, a health care consulting firm specializing in Medicare reimbursement and coding. Mrs. Rose has extensive knowledge of past and present Medicare regulations and is devoted to assisting ophthalmology practices in understanding and implementing those regulations. She also conducts coding lectures for numerous ophthalmology societies and is a member of the American Society of Ophthalmic Administrators (ASOA). Mrs. Rose is editor and publisher of *The Messenger*, a newsletter written and developed specifically for the specialty of ophthalmology, and is also on the Board of Advisors for the *Ophthalmology Compliance & Reimbursement Insider*.

Heather B. Freeland is director of coding and compliance for Rose & Associates and has over 30 years experience in the health care industry. Heather served as a Medicare fair hearing officer for 8 years prior to joining Rose & Associates. Her professional career began in the Medicare division at Blue Cross and Blue Shield of Texas where she worked in reimbursement, quality assurance auditing and post-payment medical review. She also was responsible for answering congressional inquiries from federal legislators.

Heather is very familiar with Medicare legislation, regulations ,and instructions from the Centers for Medicare & Medicaid Services. She is available to assist clients with responses to audit requests, preparing, and handling fair hearings and administrative law judge hearings, as well as conducting practice chart audits for compliance.

She currently authors the reimbursement section of "In Your Practice," which appears regularly in the *American Society of Ophthalmic Administrators (ASOA) Administrative Eyecare* magazine, and contributes regularly to *Ophthalmology Compliance & Reimbursement Insider*, *Ophthalmology Management*, and *Review of Ophthalmology*.

Kevin Corcoran, COE, CPC, FNAO is president and co-owner of Corcoran Consulting Group in Southern California. His company provides ophthalmologists, optometrists, opticians, hospitals, ambulatory surgery centers, and manufacturers with assistance on Medicare, Medicaid, and other third-party reimbursement problems.

Prior to starting his business with his wife Sue in 1985, he spent over 10 years in ophthalmology in a variety of sales and marketing positions, most recently as marketing information manager and reimbursement specialist for IOLAB Corporation. Kevin is also a registered optician and contact lens technician and enjoys the added perspective that clinical practice offers.

He received his bachelor of science degree in biology from the University of California at Irvine in 1974. He attended the Graduate School of Business at California State University, San Francisco, with an emphasis in finance and marketing.

Kevin became a certified procedural coder by the American Academy of Professional Coders in December 1999. He has also obtained the certified ophthalmic executive designation from the American Society of Ophthalmic Administrators (ASOA) in the spring of 1999.

Sue Corcoran, COE is vice president and cofounder of Corcoran Consulting Group in Southern California. She has an extensive background in medical office management and accounts receivable management, starting as a receptionist and medical assistant in 1969.

Her background also includes sales and marketing positions with manufacturers of medical devices. Sue also owned and operated a medical billing service, which specialized in ophthalmic practices for 12 years, until its sale in 1997. Sue enjoys visiting client practices and helping to identify and resolve problems.

Mary Pat Johnson, COMT, CPC, COE has been in the field of ophthalmology since 1987. She began her career as an ophthalmic technician with the Spokane Eye Clinic. Her most recent clinical position was with the department of ophthalmology at Loma Linda University, Loma Linda, Calif, as a nursing/clinic supervisor.

In 1990, she received Joint Commission on Allied Health Personnel in Ophthalmology (JCAHPO) certification as an ophthalmic technologist. She successfully completed the professional coders certification (CPC) through the American Academy of Professional Coders in 1999, and the certified ophthalmic executive status through the ASOA in spring 2001. Mary Pat has been with Corcoran Consulting Group since 1992.

Mary Pat continues to teach continuing education and workshops locally and at national and regional meetings.

Patricia J. Kennedy, COMT, COE, CPC has been in the field of ophthalmology since 1985. She began her career as a receptionist, billing clerk, and ophthalmic assistant for Dr. Tom Gillette in Seattle, Wash. In 1990, she received her certification as an ophthalmic technologist.

Her most recent clinical position was at Pacific Northwest Eye Associates in Tacoma, Wash, as a clinic supervisor, where she was charged with improving documentation and coding in accordance with new and ever evolving HCFA guidelines.

Because of her growing interest in this area, she recently became an associate with Corcoran Consulting Group. She continues to maintain her certification in the clinical aspects of ophthalmology. Patricia also became a certified procedural coder by the American Academy of Professional Coders in December 2001.

Linda Georgian, COE has been working with eye care professionals since 1985. Her experience includes project planning and implementation of several information systems, accounts receivable management for large groups and ASCs, managed care contracting, optical management, and administration. She has also facilitated start-up Laser Vision Correction programs for two general ophthalmology clinics.

Linda has had extensive exposure to large practice mergers and how to manage business operations while working with the Inland Eye Institute Medical Group, Inc, Palm Desert, Calif. Notably, she has been in charge of, and participated in, three information system purchases and installations throughout her career.

She excels in project planning, design, and coordination, with an emphasis on increased productivity and enhanced efficiency. She received her certification as a certified ophthalmic executive in the spring of 2001.

Donna McCune, CCS-P, COE is a senior consultant with Corcoran Consulting Group in Southern California. Prior to joining the Consulting Group, she was an administrator in a high-volume medical/surgical ophthalmic practice in Connecticut for 12 years.

Her responsibilities included strategic planning, financial reporting, marketing, and personnel. An active member with the American Society of Ophthalmic Administrators, she served on the ASOA Board of Governors from 1997 to 1998 and is currently serving on the ASOA Certification Board.

McCune received her certification as a certified coding specialist for physicians from the American Health Information Management Association in the fall of 1998 and certified ophthalmic executive certification in the spring of 1999.

Allison Weber Shuren, MSN, JD has focused her practice on regulatory and legislative health care matters involving corporate compliance programs and reviews, Medicare and Medicaid reimbursement, fraud and abuse counseling, practitioner licensure, and health insurance issues. She currently advises a diverse group of clients, including hospitals, physician practices, nursing specialty societies, and ambulatory surgery centers.

Prior to attending law school, Ms. Shuren was in practice as a critical care clinical nurse specialist and certified pediatric nurse practitioner at a major academic children's medical center. In this capacity, Ms. Shuren was responsible not only for clinical care of patients, but was also involved in the institution's development of an outcomes management and interdisciplinary clinical pathway program for managed care contracting. Ms. Shuren has given numerous invited presentations to both nursing associations and medical groups on a wide range of health care topics, as well as authored several peer-reviewed articles and a book chapter.

Ms. Shuren attended University of Michigan Law School where she specialized in health care law and the Employee Retirement Income Security Act. She also worked for the University of Michigan Medical Center Attorney's Office and the Michigan Governor's Commission on Genetic Privacy. During an internship at the US Food and Drug Administration Office of International

Policy, Ms. Shuren focused on harmonization of international pharmaceutical and medical device standards.

Bill Sarraille, JD is a member of the Health Care Practice Group at the Washington, DC and New York, NY law firm of Arent, Fox, Kintner, Plotkin, & Kahn. Mr. Sarraille concentrates on a variety of health care matters, including Stark Law and anti-kickback analyses, Medicare and Medicaid audits and overpayment issues, compliance program audits and installations, physician compensation issues, acquisitions, managed care matters, transactional and contract projects, administrative litigation, legislative matters, Part B reimbursement issues, Health Insurance Portability and Accountability Act (HIPAA) privacy and security issues, clinical research issues, and the defense of health care criminal and False Claims Act matters. Mr. Sarraille also represents a number of health care trade associations and serves as national regulatory councel to the Ophthalmic Mutual Insurance Company (OMIC).

Mr. Sarraille served as a law clerk to the Honorable Harry L. Hupp in the US District Court for the Central District of California in Los Angeles in 1989 and 1990. He is a member of the Bar of the District of Columbia and the state of California. He is admitted to the Bars of the US Court of Appeals for the District of Columbia and the Fourth, Sixth, and Ninth Circuits. Mr. Sarraille is also admitted to a number of the Bars of the US District Courts. He is a member of the Healthcare Financial Management Association, the National Health Lawyers Association, and the Health Care Compliance Association. He is a member of the American Hospital Association's Regulatory Relief Committee.

Jeffrey Peters, JD currently advises a diverse group of clients on a wide range of health care issues, focusing on fraud and abuse counseling, health care business transactions, state and federal regulatory compliance, and Medicare reimbursement issues. Mr. Peters has particular expertise in the application of the federal Anti-Kickback Statute and the federal Physician Self-Referral Law to health business transactions. In addition, Mr. Peters advises ophthalmology and ambulatory surgical center related trade associations on a variety of regulatory and legislative issues.

Mr. Peters has counseled businesses and investors contemplating financial arrangements with a wide range of health care companies, conducted regulatory due diligence in connection with significant transactions, and assisted in the initial public offering of a practice management company. Mr. Peters has advised health care systems and elder care providers on the establishment of assisted living and independent living facilities, assisted clients with the federal and state regulatory issues concerning the establishment of ambulatory surgical centers, and counseled clients regarding the sale and management of physician practices to or by physician practice management companies.

Mr. Peters joined Arent Fox in 1998 after 2 years in the Health Care Practice Group of Winston & Strawn's Washington, DC office.

INTRODUCTION

A few years ago a new word appeared in the lexicon of health care regulation: *Compliance*. Spurred on by increasingly aggressive enforcement activity by federal and state governments, as well as by private payors, physicians and providers have been seeking new ways to protect themselves from allegations that they have acted inappropriately. Virtually every physician and provider in health care today strives to comply with applicable rules and regulations in order "to do the right thing"—if they could only figure out what is the right thing.

This book will not provide the answers to all of the questions that face ophthalmologists in order to help them do the right thing. If it fulfills its mission, however, it will provide information about some of the more common coding, risk management, and legal issues that face ophthalmology practices today and will provide advice on how to address those issues. Ophthalmologists are cautioned: the information in this book does not constitute legal advice, nor does it constitute coding advice. It simply serves to alert ophthalmologists to legal and coding issues that may be applicable to them. Any specific questions should be directed to one's lawyer or coding consultant.

The contributors to this book have extensive experience working with ophthalmology practices, and some of us have done so for more than 20 years. Each of us has enormous respect for the profession and for the clients with whom we have had the privilege to work. This book reflects a compilation of the most common issues we have identified over the course of our work. If every reader finds at least one issue that applies to his or her practice and helps to bring that practice closer to full compliance, then we will consider the hours spent developing this book to have been most worthwhile.

—*Alan Reider, MPH, JD*

REIMBURSEMENT ISSUES

1

NEW PATIENT FOR THE PHYSICIAN OR NEW PATIENT FOR THE PRACTICE?

A physician joins a new group practice and does not bring patient medical records from his prior practice. One of the physician's prior, established patients is scheduled for an annual diabetic check in the new practice. Prior to the examination, a new patient chart is created, medical history obtained, patient demographic information form completed, and lifetime signature statement obtained.

IS THIS SERVICE CONSIDERED AN ESTABLISHED PATIENT VISIT OR MAY A NEW PATIENT VISIT BE BILLED?

Medicare interprets the phrase "new patient" to mean a patient who has not received any professional services from the physician within the previous 3 years.

Therefore, if the same physician in the prior practice saw the patient within the past 3 years, a new patient examination would not be appropriate. In this case, the physician may bill a level of "established office visit" code to reflect the time and effort necessary to review the patient's medical history, data and tests, and physical examination required since this information was not available to the new practice.

However, had the patient received only technical services such as pressure checks, contact lens fittings, renewal of prescriptions, etc, and had no face-to-face encounter with the physician in the last 3 years, then the "new patient" visit may be coded. Technical services do not constitute "physician professional services," and documentation of these types of services in the patient chart would not prohibit a physician from billing a new patient examination.

MISIDENTIFICATION OF THE PROVIDER

A group of ophthalmologists added an optometrist to the practice. The optometrist assisted the ophthalmologists by working up their patients. Those patients who did not have the need to see an ophthalmologist were examined and treated by the optometrist. For the purpose of reimbursement, no one in the practice bothered to enroll the optometrist as a member of the group in any insurance plans. An ophthalmologist within the group evaluated all of the optometrist's charts and countersigned them as acceptable. The group then used that ophthalmologist's name and personal identification number (PIN) for billing all insurance companies, even though the ophthalmologist did not render the service.

IS THIS PROCESS ACCEPTABLE TO MEDICARE AND OTHER PAYORS?

This process is not acceptable under Medicare requirements or those of any other insurance company. Each physician (eg, ophthalmologist or optometrist) in a group practice must apply for and maintain his or her own identification number. That number must be reflected on the claim form to identify who provided the service.

By way of example, one Medicare carrier addresses the issue of improper use of another physician's PIN as follows:

> Connecticut Medicare is also aware that some groups or entities are submitting claims for the new physicians or non-physician practitioners using one of the other physician's Medicare Provider Identification numbers while waiting for the new PIN to be issued. This is not acceptable practice. Before these services can be billed to Medicare, each provider must obtain his or her own PIN. The claims for that provider should be held until Medicare issues a PIN number.

It is important to recognize that the delay in obtaining a PIN will not likely impact the ability of the physician or practice to be paid for the services. The Medicare program and most insurers will accept claims for services rendered starting with the date the PIN request was submitted. Thus, while waiting for the issuance of a PIN may create temporary cash flow problems, it should not adversely affect payment. On the other hand, to use an incorrect PIN to obtain payment could result in allegations that an improper claim was submitted with potentially severe penalties.

3

BILLING CONSULTATIONS
WITHIN A GROUP PRACTICE

A cataract surgeon sees a patient for an annual intraocular lens (IOL) examination. The patient is diabetic and complains of decreased vision. A dilated, comprehensive eye examination reveals normal anterior segment with capsules open and diabetic retinopathy with suspicious lesions. The cataract surgeon suggests that the patient see a retina specialist within the group as soon as possible. The *Plan* entry of the patient's chart indicates "Referred to retina specialist for diabetic retinopathy eval; return in 1 year for IOL check."

Upon returning to the front desk to schedule the retinal appointment, the patient learns that the retina doctor is available immediately and proceeds to the retina doctor's office.

The technician indicates "Referred by Dr. X for diabetic retinal eval" in the *Subjective* entry of the chart. The retinal doctor reviews the findings in the earlier examination and decides to repeat the fundus examination, perform an extended ophthalmoscopy, and then orders a fluorescein angiogram (FA). The results of the retina evaluation and diagnostic tests are noted in the chart. The patient is diagnosed with diabetic retinopathy with no active lesions. No treatment is necessary for the old lesions that were causing the decreased vision, and the patient is told to return in 6 months for a follow-up exam or to call immediately if the symptoms worsen.

The patient chart is then returned to the cataract surgeon to review the findings of the retina evaluation. The cataract surgeon initials the findings in the patient's chart as read.

IS THE INTRAOFFICE CONSULTATION BILLABLE?

One of the most common billing errors in ophthalmology is the failure to bill for intraoffice consultations within a group practice. Referrals for evaluation between two different specialty trained physicians within the same clinic can establish the basis for a consultation. The documentation that is required to support an intraoffice consultation is the same as a regular consultation, with the exception that a separate written report, beyond the consultant's entry in the practice's medical record, does not need to be furnished to the referring physician.

The consultant's report that is already a part of the patient's medical record can serve as the written report of findings. It is recommended that the referring physician review and initial the findings.

Caution should be taken when billing the level of service for intraoffice consultations. Since the patient has already been examined by another ophthalmologist and is being referred for a specific problem within the ocular system, the highest level that can normally be justified is an Expanded Problem Focused office consultation (code 99242). In many cases, only a Problem Focused office consultation (code 99241) would be justified.

The level of service billed must comply with all the documentation requirements of history, examination, and medical decision making. There also must be documented evidence of the need for the level of service billed, which will be based on the nature of the patient's presenting problem.

VISUAL FIELD TESTING
FOR GLAUCOMA PATIENTS

An established patient with advanced glaucoma returns to the office only for a visual field test. During the previous 3-month glaucoma check, the physician observed some changes on the optic nerve fiber and ordered the visual field to be performed today, since the patient could not stay for the test at the prior visit. This is the fifth visual field the patient has had this year, and the billing staff asks whether it is billable.

ARE THERE ANY GUIDELINES TO LET US KNOW HOW OFTEN A VISUAL FIELD CAN BE BILLED TO MEDICARE IN A 12 MONTH PERIOD?

Carrier frequency parameters are considered proprietary by Medicare and not generally released to the public. However, some Medicare carriers have begun to publish Local Medical Review Policies (LMRPs), indicating what would be considered medically necessary for billing visual fields.

In lieu of any published carrier guidelines, physicians must rely on their own medical expertise to determine how often to bill for certain diagnostic tests. For support, physicians may refer to the American Academy of Ophthalmology's Preferred Practice Patterns (PPP) for treating glaucoma patients. The PPP-suggested frequency parameters for medically necessary visual fields for glaucoma patients are as follows:

Compliant Patient With No Progression of Damage to the Optic Nerve

✧ Six months after the initial visual fields
✧ Every 12 to 24 months

Noncompliant Patient With Progressive Damage to the Optic Nerve

✧ Every 6 to 12 months, with no noticeable changes in the visual fields voiced by the patient

✧ Every 3 to 6 months when the patient reports changes in his or her visual fields or the physician notes changes in the eye during the examination to suggest possible visual field loss such as significant changes in the optic disc

Advanced Glaucoma Patient

✧ Every 3 months in patients with advanced glaucoma

Physicians should be certain to determine whether their carrier has published a specific LMRP for visual fields; if so, physicians must follow those specific guidelines.

5

SCANNING LASER GLAUCOMA TEST

A practice has purchased a new piece of scanning laser equipment that is designed to help in the early detection of glaucoma. In the past, the practice always billed for a visual field and fundus photos. Now that the practice is using the new GDX Nerve Fiber Analyzer (GDX), the practice seems to be performing the test on every patient who has a family history of glaucoma and not simply on its established glaucoma patients. In addition, a question arises whether the practice should be billing this procedure as a "per eye" or as a unilateral service.

WHAT ARE THE GUIDELINES FOR BILLING SCANNING LASER EQUIPMENT TO MEDICARE?

The scanning laser test (eg, GDX, Heidelberg Retina Tomograph, etc) allows for earlier detection of glaucoma damage to the nerve fiber layer or optic nerve of the eye. It is the goal of these glaucoma diagnostic tests to discriminate among patients with normal intraocular pressures (IOP) who have glaucoma, patients with elevated IOP who have glaucoma, and patients with elevated IOP who do not have glaucoma. This allows early treatment of the disease, preventing unnecessary medical or surgical therapy.

Most carriers have published specific billing guidelines for code 92135 that generally include the following protocols:

- ✧ The scanning laser glaucoma test is used once a year to follow preglaucoma patients (elevated IOP but no signs of glaucoma) or those with "mild damage to the nerve fiber layer."
- ✧ Patients with "moderate damage" may be followed with both scanning laser glaucoma test and visual fields. One or two of each test per year may be appropriate.
- ✧ In "advanced damage," visual field testing would be preferred instead of scanning laser glaucoma tests. Most carriers believe

that it is rarely necessary to perform more than four visual fields in a year in "advanced damage," and scanning laser glaucoma tests are rarely necessary or beneficial.

Code 92135 is billable as a unilateral service (ie, per eye). In addition, a physician's order must be recorded in the chart, and a separate interpretation and report must be included. The printout of the scanning laser results usually have a "comments" section that can be used to document the report by the physician.

Most carriers will deny the following procedures if performed on the same day as the scanning laser, unless medical necessity for the additional tests is clearly noted in the chart:

✧ Fundus Photos (92250)

✧ Extended Ophthalmoscopy (92225 and 92226)

✧ B-Scan (76512)

Physicians should always check their Medicare newsletters for specific billing guidelines.

6

EXAMINATION PERFORMED THE SAME DAY AS ARGON LASER TRABECULOPASTY

A patient presents for a 3-month glaucoma check and states "frequently forgets to use glaucoma drops." The patient's intraocular pressure (IOP) is chronically at 22, which is above the target pressure of 12. The patient is on maximum medication but is unable to comply with using the drops. After a complete examination, the doctor determines that the patient would benefit from laser surgery since the patient has difficulty complying with the use of the glaucoma medications. The patient agrees and is taken to the laser room for an argon laser trabeculoplasty (ALT).

IS THE VISIT BILLABLE WHEN A SURGICAL PROCEDURE WAS PERFORMED THE SAME DAY?

An office visit on the same day as a minor surgery (0 or 10 day global fee period) is included in the payment for the surgery unless a significant, separately identifiable service also is performed that requires the use of the 25 modifier.

With the global fee period for argon laser trabeculoplasty (code 65855) reduced from 90 days to 10 days, the ALT is considered a "minor" surgical procedure. As such, any examination performed on the same day must be documented as a separately identifiable examination in order to justify a separate bill.

Since the physician did not determine until the end of the examination that surgery was needed, the modifier 25 would be appropriate. Had the patient presented for the ALT, and the physician examined only the angles and performed an IOP check, the visit would not have been separately billable.

GLAUCOMA SCREENING EXAM

A patient presents for an annual cataract check for incipient cataracts. The patient's history sheet shows that the patient's mother had glaucoma. As part of a dilated comprehensive eye examination, the patient's intraocular pressure (IOP) is checked, a fundus examination is performed, and the anterior chamber is examined. The patient's pressure is found to be within normal limits, angles are open, and the optic nerve and disc are healthy and pink. The patient's cataracts have not progressed, but the patient requires new glasses to correct the vision. The doctor recommends a return in 1 year for a cataract check.

Six months later, the patient calls the office indicating he read in *Modern Maturity* that Medicare covers an eye examination for glaucoma screening. Since the patient's mother had glaucoma, the patient asks to be scheduled for a glaucoma screening examination.

WHAT ARE THE REQUIREMENTS FOR BILLING THE NEW GLAUCOMA SCREENING EXAMINATION, AND WOULD THIS PATIENT BE ELIGIBLE TO RECEIVE THIS NEW COVERED BENEFIT?

Medicare covers an annual glaucoma screening examination for patients with diabetes mellitus, patients who have a family history of glaucoma, and African-Americans age 50 and over who are Medicare eligible. The procedure code is Glaucoma screening furnished by an optometrist or ophthalmologist (G0117). The diagnosis code is V80.1, Special screening for neurological, eye, and ear diseases; glaucoma. Screening examinations submitted with any other diagnosis will be automatically denied.

Medicare defines the term "screening for glaucoma" as (1) a dilated eye examination with an IOP measurement, and (2) a direct ophthalmoscopy or a slit-lamp examination. The glaucoma screening examination cannot be billed in conjunction with any other examination. In fact, Medicare believes that physicians will more commonly provide glaucoma tests in conjunction with other services and will rarely provide only glaucoma screening to Medicare patients.

In this scenario, the glaucoma screening benefit would not be allowed since the patient received a glaucoma screening as part of his annual cataract evaluation. If the patient had not received any other glaucoma screening service in the prior 11 months, then this screening examination would be billable to Medicare. To determine the 11-month period, count begins with the month after the month in which the previous covered screening procedure was performed.

8

INTERPRETATION AND REPORTS FOR DIAGNOSTIC TESTS

A patient presents for an annual diabetic examination and complains of a slight decrease in vision. Upon examination, the patient's best-corrected visual acuity has decreased from 20/30 to 20/60. The physician performs a dilated, comprehensive eye examination, as defined by Medicare, and observes that a few lesions are now present in the macula.

A fluorescein angiogram (FA) and fundus photos are ordered. Upon review of the films, the physician determines that the patient needs a focal laser treatment.

WHAT DOCUMENTATION IS REQUIRED TO SUPPORT THE SERVICES PROVIDED?

The physician must first identify the most generally accepted content of the interpretation and report. The written entry should answer the following questions:

✧ *Why is the test being performed?* Give the questionable symptoms or the medical condition being followed. In the above scenario, the interpretation and report of both the FA and fundus photos should indicate that both tests are being performed to determine the source of the macular hemorrhage.

✧ *What was found and were the results as expected or were there new findings?* The interpretation of the FA should indicate "new hemorrhage, subfoveal of the choroidal layer, etc." The interpretation of the fundus photo should document the specific location of the hemorrhage as well as any other anomalies.

✧ *Finally, how do the results affect the treatment of the patient's medical condition?* Both tests must indicate "focal laser" as a plan of treatment.

The reason for the test should be the same as the diagnosis used to bill the test. Remember that the results do not dictate the reason for the test. It is the medical condition, sign, or symptom that dictates the medical necessity for the test. The reason for the test should be easily identified in the chart, either outright in the order for the test, or in the body of the examination findings.

The interpreting physician should record the results of the test in a conspicuous area of the chart, on the actual printout, or in a separate interpretation and report. If the test is a photo that is stored on film or in a computer, the location of the photos must be clearly noted in the chart. Finally, these test results must be easily retrievable in the event of an audit.

9

DIAGNOSIS CODING

In an effort to consolidate its billing functions, a large group practice with several satellite locations centralized its billing office at one location. The route slips (or superbills) were completed by the physicians and staff and couriered to the billing office for data entry and claim submission. The billing office staff relied on the route slips to bill the service provided, the level of service, and appropriate diagnosis codes. Many of the routing slips contained three or more diagnosis codes. The billing staff listed all the diagnosis codes on the claims.

How Does Diagnosis Coding Influence Reimbursement?

The proper use of diagnosis codes (ICD-9) serves as the mechanism to advise a payor the reason a particular procedure or service was performed. Use of an improper ICD-9 code can result in a payment for a service that is not covered or denial of a payment for a service that should be covered.

The primary diagnosis should be consistent with the reason for the patient's visit or reflect the chief complaint. For example, a Medicare patient presents for an exam stating he recently broke his glasses and needs a new prescription. He reports no difficulty with his vision. The exam reveals very early nuclear sclerosis, and his best-corrected vision is 20/20 in both eyes. The appropriate primary diagnosis for this patient is presbyopia because it is consistent with the reason for his visit. This service should be noncovered by Medicare regardless of the fact that a diagnosis of cataracts was made.

The *Medicare Carriers Manual*, Part 3 §2320 reads:

> The coverage of services rendered by an ophthalmologist is dependent on the purpose of the examination rather than on

the ultimate diagnosis of the patient's condition. When a beneficiary goes to an ophthalmologist with a complaint or symptoms of an eye disease or injury, the ophthalmologist's services (except for eye refractions) are covered regardless of the fact that only eyeglasses were prescribed. However, when a beneficiary goes to his or her ophthalmologist for an eye examination with no specific complaint, the expenses for the examination are not covered even though as a result of such examination the doctor discovered a pathologic condition.

If a biller erroneously listed cataract as the basis for the visit, Medicare would pay. A subsequent review of the medical record as part of a postpayment audit, however, would result in an overpayment determination, if not risking more serious sanction.

Several considerations should be made when an ICD-9 code is selected for the claim form:

✧ Be as specific as possible and consistent with the patient's medical record. The most specific ICD-9 codes have four or five digits. Using nonspecific codes may not reveal adequate medical necessity for the service.

✧ A history of the disease may be appropriate for a condition that no longer exists (eg, V-codes).

✧ Code symptoms if no definitive diagnosis can be determined. Do not describe the patient with a disease or condition he or she does not have. "Rule out" does not exist in the ICD-9 manual.

✧ Document whether the condition is chronic or acute and what the planned treatment is. If it is acute in an emergency situation, be sure to identify the nature of the condition. A chronic disease can be listed multiple times as long as it continues to be treated.

✧ Identify how injuries occurred.

✧ List chronic conditions or secondary diagnoses only if they are pertinent to that particular visit.

✧ Be consistent with CPT rules. For example, if you use a code subject to the "separate procedure" rule, then identify an additional diagnosis to justify that service.

✧ Understand the third-party payor guidelines. Some payors truncate the diagnosis list and ignore the second or third ICD-9 code.

The critical problem in this case is the failure of the biller to be able to determine the precise diagnosis code that reflected the physician's decision to provide a procedure or service. Further, the physicians continued to include diagnoses based on the patient's prior ocular history. This further confused the billers. Where physicians use billers either within their practice or contract out for such services, they must take care to ensure that the services performed and the reason for the service are clearly identified and linked on the route slip.

10

PROPERLY DOCUMENTING FUNCTIONAL BLEPHAROPLASTY SURGERY

A patient presents to the office complaining of inability to see low-lying tree limbs while out walking and also having to raise eyelids manually when trying to read street signs. Upon examination, the patient's visual acuity is 20/20 with eyelids raised by the examiner. The doctor observes that the patient's lids cover two-thirds of the pupil in the left eye and half the pupil in the right eye. The patient's lid crease measures 13 mm and the lid fissure measures 12 mm. The patient also demonstrates severe dermatochalasis by measurement and external photos.

The physician orders a visual field with the eyelids in repose, as well as in a taped position. A report documents that the patient has severe upper field loss that is corrected upon taping the eyelids. The physician discusses the findings with the patient and recommends bilateral ptosis repair with removal of the excess skin.

HAS THE CHART BEEN PROPERLY DOCUMENTED TO SUBSTANTIATE BILLING MEDICARE FOR A FUNCTIONAL REPAIR OF THE EYELID?

Documenting the medical necessity of lid surgery, mainly blepharoplasty for the repair of blepharochalasis or dermatochalasis, is extremely difficult. Medicare and other third-party payors generally take the position that the excision of excess skin is cosmetic. While it may be apparent to the physician that the procedure will provide an improvement of the patient's visual difficulty, payors must be able to follow the physician's thought process on paper in the event of audit.

To develop the necessary documentation, physicians must record, in detail, the patient's lifestyle problems with the "droopy lid." As with all patient complaints, this should be documented in the patient's own words and in quotes. In addition, the record should include preoperative photographs (at least two copies). Most Medicare carriers no longer require the photographs to be submitted in advance with the claim, but physicians must have a second set available in the event Medicare develops the claim for additional information. Always obtain preoperative visual fields (ie, tangent screen, 78-point screen, or 80-point screen) with the lid taped up and with the lid in normal position. Since this results in two isopter fields, the maximum billable level of visual fields would be code 92082, Intermediate visual field.

The external photos and the visual fields are required for medical necessity and are reimbursable by Medicare. Physicians should resist any attempt by the payor to deny the external photos; appeal the denials since the photos are a carrier requirement and not a routine part of the exam.

It is also important to understand that medical necessity will not be supported by the documentation of the patient's visual acuity without the lid problem. If the patient is 20/20 without any significant visual field loss documented in the chart, the question to be considered is whether the procedure is cosmetic or functional. If this procedure can help the patient functionally, then proceed after you have documented the medical necessity, medical justification, and medical reasonableness of the procedure in the patient's chart.

BILLING OFFICE VISITS THE
SAME DAY AS MAJOR SURGERY

A patient presents to the physician with a complaint of decreased vision after a satisfactory cataract surgery 9 months earlier. The patient states that oncoming headlights while driving causes glare again. The best-corrected visual acuity is 20/25, but vision decreases to 20/40 on glare testing. The doctor examines the patient and determines that 2+ posterior capsule opacification exists and a YAG laser capsulotomy is indicated. The patient is taken to the laser room and the YAG is performed before the patient leaves the office.

MAY THE PHYSICIAN BILL FOR THE EXAMINATION PERFORMED ON THE SAME DAY AS SURGERY?

Office visits by the same physician on the day before or the same day as a major surgery (ie, within the 90-day global fee period) are included in the payment for the procedure, unless the visit establishes the decision to perform the surgery. In this case, the visit on the day of surgery was properly documented as the visit to determine the need for surgery; therefore, the visit may be billed to Medicare with a –57 modifier, reflecting an evaluation and management service that resulted in the decision to perform surgery.

12

MISCODING AND FRAGMENTATION OF RETINAL LASER SURGERY

A patient presented with ocular manifestation of diabetes in both eyes, including diabetic macular edema and proliferative diabetic retinopathy. After thorough examination, the physician planned laser treatment to the right eye to begin the same day. Similar treatment to the left eye is planned for the near future. The patient consented to "argon focal laser and initial panretinal photocoagulation (PRP), right eye." The operative report indicated 89 laser spots were applied around the macula, and an additional 490 spots were applied in the peripheral retina of the right eye. The office submitted a claim for only the focal laser (code 67210). When the patient returned 2 weeks later, an additional 270 laser spots were applied to the peripheral retina of the right eye and a claim was submitted for argon laser PRP (code 67288).

WERE THESE SERVICES BILLED APPROPRIATELY?

No. The initial claim identified the service as focal treatment when PRP was actually performed as well. In this instance, where laser is both applied in the macular region as well as the periphery, the term "panretinal" applies to the entire treatment even though the physician was addressing two different aspects of the diabetic disease: diabetic macular edema and proliferative diabetic retinopathy. The correct coding for the initial date of service is 67228 (PRP). The CPT book contains the phrase "one or more sessions" as part of the definition for PRP and a number of other laser procedures. When PRP is performed in stages, only the initial procedure is reimbursed. Thus, the session performed 2 weeks later was ineligible for reimbursement.

The confusion surrounding the billing for the initial laser treatment arose because the operative report stated "argon focal laser and initial PRP." The physician performed focal laser for macular edema as well as PRP for proliferative diabetic retinopathy during the same operative session. This problem can be eliminated if the argon focal is performed on a separate day from the initial PRP setting. When both procedures occur within the global period (90 days for retinal laser procedure), the subsequent claim requires modifier −79.

13

An established patient with previously diagnosed glaucoma presents to the office for a scheduled glaucoma check. The patient has no complaints, but when the technician takes the patient's pressure, the pressure is documented as 30 mmHg. The patient admits to not using drops for a month and a half. The physician is then called in to see the patient and subsequently performs a slit lamp examination and administers Iopidine (Alcon, Fort Worth, TX), to lower the pressure. The doctor also spends a considerable amount of time advising the patient of the need for regular adherence to using the glaucoma drops.

IS A MORE EXTENSIVE EVALUATION AND MANAGEMENT (E/M) SERVICE BILLABLE OR MAY THE PHYSICIAN BILL ONLY FOR THE DOCUMENTED BRIEF SERVICE?

Normally, this examination would be billed as a Problem-focused, established patient visit (code 99212). However, on rare occasions it may be necessary for the physician to spend more than 50% of the total exam time face-to-face with the patient counseling on such issues as:

1. Giving diagnostic results, impressions, and/or recommended diagnostic studies
2. Discussing prognosis
3. Discussing risks and benefits of treatment options
4. Giving instructions for treatment and/or follow-up
5. Discussing the importance of compliance with chosen treatment options
6. How to reduce risk factors

When this occurs, time may be used as a factor in choosing the level of service as long as the time spent on counseling and the topic(s) discussed are documented in the patient chart. For example, if the total examination lasted for 25 minutes and the physician spent 15 minutes of that visit in face-to-face counseling with the patient, the visit may usually be increased to a Level 3 E/M service (code 99213). Documentation required includes the start and finish time of the entire examination and the breakdown of the examination and counseling should be shown (eg, 10-minute exam, 15 minutes counseling the patient on the importance of using the prescribed glaucoma drops).

Face-to-face applies to *physician face-to-face time only*. Time spent with the technician cannot be included in the time factor.

14

BILLING FOR NEW TECHNOLOGY

A busy retina specialist attended several conferences to learn more about the emerging techniques and technology used to treat age-related macular degeneration (AMD). During the lectures, he heard a leading retina specialist tout the merits of these new procedures. The speaker mentioned that there is an existing CPT code that describes these procedures and encouraged billing with this code. The retina specialist was enthused by what he heard in the courses and visited the vendor's booth to inquire about purchasing the instruments and subsequent reimbursement. The vendors assured him that the existing CPT code could be used to bill for these procedures. The retina specialist purchased the instrument and began treating patients with AMD.

DOES THE FACT THAT A CPT CODE APPLIES TO THE PROCEDURE ENSURE PAYMENT?

The existence of a CPT code does not ensure reimbursement or coverage of a surgical procedure. In this case, third-party payors might deem the "new" technology unproven, experimental, or investigational. Payors generally are suspicious of procedures for which there are few peer-reviewed, published articles in reputable scientific journals. Payment for such procedures is customarily the patient's responsibility. Under Medicare's program standards, investigational procedures are not covered.

The retina specialist has two problems:

1. Any paid claims may subsequently be reversed and payors require a refund
2. Pending claims will probably be denied.

Prior to making an investment in the new equipment, the physician should inquire about the position of Medicare carriers or other third-party payors with respect to the coverage of the new technology.

If a favorable coverage policy is absent, and the physician offers the procedure to a patient who may benefit from it, he should inform the patient in advance that the procedure might not be covered. Before the procedure can be performed the patient should accept financial responsibility and sign an advanced beneficiary notice.

Additionally, the physician may wish to seek the assistance of his professional society to initiate a dialogue with payers to obtain future coverage of the new procedure.

MEDICARE BILLING ISSUES
FOR AN OPTICAL DISPENSARY

In 2001, Dr. A set up an optical dispensary in his waiting room. He and his patients have been very happy with the convenience, and the optician is skilled at fitting just the right pair of glasses for each patient. While commercial insurance and self-pay revenues have been fine, Medicare has denied each claim submitted for post-cataract surgery spectacles.

WHY WAS THERE NO MEDICARE PAYMENT?

Billing Medicare for postcataract surgery glasses can be more difficult than one would anticipate. In this case, the computer billing system has been printing Dr. A's provider number for the local Medicare carrier, rather than the supplier number issued by the durable medical equipment regional contractor (DMERC) carrier, on some of the claim forms. This alone caused most of the claim rejections.

Second, since the glasses were dispensed in the doctor's office, the billing staff never thought to question the place of service. Postcataract eyeglasses, however, are paid under Medicare's prosthetic device benefit, for use by the patient at home, and "home" is the correct place of service (POS 12). This also caused claims to reject.

Third, coding turned out to be the most difficult problem. Medicare has some unusual modifier rules for DMERC claims, including those indicating medical necessity or lack thereof. For example, Medicare does not cover all features of eyeglasses. Some features are provided for cosmetic reasons or for extra convenience but are not medically necessary in the strict sense. The prescription in the lenses and a standard frame to hold them are medically necessary, but tints (V274x), photochromic lenses (V2744), oversize lenses (V2780), antireflective coatings (V2750), and polycarbonate lenses (V2730) are rarely covered. Explicit documentation of medical necessity in the physician's chart is necessary to justify reimbursement for these added features.

When an item is supplied for cosmetic reasons, such as some tints, or for convenience, antireflective coating, or photochromic lenses, then the Medicare beneficiary may pay for the "extras." During 2001, in order for these claims to be properly denied, a –ZY modifier needed to be appended to the HCPCS code. The –ZY modifier notified the DMERC that a denial was sought. The beneficiary signed an advance beneficiary notice (ABN) to indicate that he or she understood that Medicare will not pay for cosmetic or convenience items. Modifier –GA was also added to the claim line to indicate that the signed form is on file and that the patient had accepted financial responsibility for the service. Where an ABN is not obtained, the physician is prohibited from billing a patient. To the extent that a patient has been billed, refunds must be made.

Effective January 1, 2002, CMS issued new instructions concerning the life of modifiers as applied to these circumstances. As of this writing, precise application of the modifiers is unclear. Readers are urged to contact your appropriate DMERC or coding consultant for clarification.

Other common billing issues relating to optical services include:

✧ Failing to use the correct lens code
✧ Failing to maintain a proof of delivery that is signed by the patient
✧ Filing the claim on the date the glasses were ordered, rather than the date they were delivered

16

BUNDLING

In July 2001, an ophthalmologist received a request from Medicare for copies of medical records supporting previously paid claims for codes 66984 (Cataract surgery with intraocular lens) and 65875 (Severing adhesions of anterior segment of eye, incisional technique; posterior synechiae). The charts requested were for services rendered over a 5-month period in 1999. The audit resulted in denials for the services and an overpayment request. In the opinion of Medicare's reviewer, the charge for 65875 was unjustified and should have been denied as an incidental component of cataract surgery (ie, bundled under the national Correct Coding Initiative, or CCI).

WAS THE MEDICARE CARRIER DETERMINATION ACCURATE?

The Center for Medicare and Medicaid Services (CMS) developed the national CCI to promote correct coding methodologies. CCI edits are based on coding conventions defined in the American Medical Association's *Current Procedural Terminology Manual*, current standards of medical and surgical coding practice, input from specialty societies, and analysis of current coding practices. The edits are updated quarterly with an effective date of the first of every quarter (ie, January 1, April 1, July 1, and October 1). It is important to note that the edits are not retroactive but effective from the designated date.

In this case, the Medicare reviewer applied current CCI edits retroactively to prior dates of service. Specifically, code 65875 was not bundled with 66984 until July 1, 2001. As a result, the ophthalmologist pursued an appeal to a carrier hearing officer. On the basis of the improper retroactive application of the CCI edit, the hearing officer reversed the denial and overpayment determination.

Practices should be aware of the requirements of the CCI when billing for services rendered. Practices also should be aware that the CCI limitations apply prospectively only. If a carrier improperly applies a CCI edit retroactively, the practice should object and pursue its right to appeal.

17

IMPROPER BILLING FOR
EXTENDED OPHTHALMOSCOPY

Dr. M, a retina specialist, received a letter from Medicare stating that her use of extended ophthalmoscopy exceeded the expected frequency when compared with her peers. Initially, this did not alarm her; both her subspecialty training and the nature of her patient base supported the fact that she performed detailed retina examinations more frequently than general ophthalmologists. Concerned about future inquires by Medicare, the practice administrator examined a sample of 50 medical records and claims for extended ophthalmoscopy. The review uncovered a general misunderstanding of these codes (92225, 92226) by the physician and billing staff. Problems existed in both documentation of the service and in billing. Several medical records in the sample contained no retinal drawing, some had very sketchy drawings of the posterior pole, while other records contained drawings labeled as "normal fundus." Additionally, the physician used only CPT code 92225; 92226 did not appear on her route slip. Finally, the practice computer system had been programmed to append modifier –50 to all claims for extended ophthalmoscopy, which meant all claims were billed as bilateral services.

WHAT PROBLEMS EXIST WITH RESPECT TO THE BILLING?

The practice had failed to follow the detailed instructions contained in the local medical review policy for extended ophthalmoscopy. Under the heading "What Is It?" the local medical review policies (LMRP) read:

> Extended ophthalmoscopy is a detailed examination and drawing that goes beyond the standard funduscopy of an office visit. Not every fundus exam qualifies as extended ophthalmoscopy. CPT states, routine ophthalmoscopy is part of general and special ophthalmologic services whenever indicated. It is a nonitemized service and is not reported separately.

This service is indicated for a wide range of posterior segment pathology when the level of examination is *greater than* that required for routine ophthalmoscopy. Extended ophthalmoscopy is reserved for serious retinal pathology. While documentation requirements vary among Medicare carriers, all carriers demand a retinal drawing. The drawing should be large enough to include sufficient detail, standard colors, and appropriate labels.

Two codes exist in CPT to identify extended ophthalmoscopy: code 92225 (Ophthalmoscopy, extended, with retinal drawing [ie, for retinal detachment, melanoma], with interpretation and report; initial) and 92226 (subsequent). No distinction is made between new and established patients. CPT 92225 is used for the *initial exam* on a particular retinal condition. Thereafter, documentation of the subsequent service (92226) should include evidence of a change in the condition (eg, worsening or progressing) that warrants a repeated examination.

Extended ophthalmoscopy is considered a unilateral service. Separate reimbursement is made for each eye when performed bilaterally. Specific patient conditions dictate whether a unilateral or bilateral service is needed. Not all claims for extended ophthalmoscopy are bilateral. While it is common practice for physicians to perform retinal exams on both eyes, if the pathology is limited to one eye, the extended ophthalmoscopy should not be billed for both eyes. Documenting a normal fundus for the fellow eye does not support a claim for extended ophthalmoscopy.

18

ARE SOME OF THE MOST COMMON COMPLIANCE ISSUES PROBLEMS IN YOUR PRACTICE?

Practice managers may not even be aware of the regulatory implications of many seemingly innocuous situations. You may want to consider how your practice would identify and deal with the following situations.

SCENARIO 1

A retinal specialty practice receives a scheduling call from a general ophthalmologist's office (Dr. Y) from which the retina group often receives referrals. The staff person from Dr. Y's office asks that the retina specialist (Dr. X) "see and evaluate the patient for Dr. Y." The patient is a Medicare patient. The chief complaint is filled out as follows: "Patient referred by Dr. Y for consultation."

The patient comes to the office and is evaluated. Dr. X orders diagnostic tests and follow-up services, as indicated by the examination. After the visit, Dr. X sends a consultation letter to Dr. Y. Dr. X's office bills the Medicare program for a consultation.

Is This a Consultation?

Was Dr. X's evaluation of the patient a *consultation*, as that term is defined by the Medicare program?

According to the Medicare program, a consultation is provided by a physician whose opinion or advice regarding the evaluation or management of a specific problem is requested by another physician or appropriate practitioner. In other words, the hallmark of a consultation is the subjective intent of the requesting physician to receive advice or an opinion. The request for the consultation and the need for the consultation must be documented in the patient's medical record. Further, the consultant must prepare a written report of his or her findings, and the report must be provided to the requesting physician or practitioner.

The Medicare program will not consider the session to be a consultation if there has been a transfer of care. A transfer of care occurs when the referring physician transfers the responsibility for the patient's complete care for the relevant problem or issue, at the time of the referral.

Applied to the situation above, many of the consultation requirements appear to be met. However, the crucial element here, as so often the case, is the intent of the requesting physician. Again, Medicare rules require that the initial physician *requests* the consultation.

In the hypothetical, the initiation came verbally from Dr. Y's office, and asked for an *evaluation*. How do we know what the initiating physician was requesting? Was it a consultation or was it simply a request for an evaluation and management or an eye code service?

Dr. Y's request was, unfortunately, ambiguous. Although Dr. Y's request for a review might be interpreted to suggest that a consultation was desired, the failure of the requesting physician's office to specifically request a *consultation*, and Dr. X's scheduler's failure to clarify the nature of the request, make the classification of this service ultimately a matter of guesswork. The chief complaint entry, despite the fact that it uses the word *consultation*, actually complicates the problem by using the term *referral*. In Medicare parlance, there is no *referral* or *referring physician* in a consultation service. Those terms are considered to be consistent only with situations where the care of the patient is transferred from the initiating physician or practitioner to another provider of care.

RISK MANAGEMENT ISSUES

Section 2

19

SECOND EYE SURGERY
BASED ON ORIGINAL EXAM

After an examination, an ophthalmologist determines that a Medicare patient is in need of cataract surgery in both eyes. It is clear to the ophthalmologist that the patient has impairment of visual function due to bilateral cataracts. At this time, the patient reports that she cannot function adequately because of decreased vision and has difficulty with several important activities of daily living, such as reading and driving. The patient's best-corrected visual acuity is 20/50 or worse in both eyes.

Based on these factors, at the conclusion of the examination, the patient is scheduled for cataract surgery in the first eye. At the first postoperative day, the patient's operated eye is examined and found to be doing well. The patient remarks how well she can see and is eager to have surgery on her second eye. Her remarks are recorded in the medical record, and she is scheduled for the second eye surgery.

WAS IT PROPER TO ORDER THE SECOND EYE
SURGERY BASED ON THE ORIGINAL EXAMINATION?

The Medicare program requires that services be *reasonable and medically necessary* in order to qualify for reimbursement. The documentation in the patient's medical record must substantiate that this standard has been met. In the case of cataract surgery, each procedure—meaning for the first eye as well as the second—must be supported by adequate documentation that justifies the medical necessity of the surgery.

In this case, the medical record supports the necessity of the surgery on the first eye. The question, however, is whether the second eye surgery is also *reasonable and medically necessary*, as those terms are used by the Medicare program.

Unfortunately, under Medicare reimbursement policy, the fellow eye procedure described on the previous page is not supported by a finding of medical necessity. According to the Medicare program, the necessity of the fellow eye procedure must be determined by a separate qualification of the second eye following the stabilization of the first eye. Thus, Medicare program reimbursement policy requires that the second eye cataract surgery be justified by independent subjective complaints from the patient. So, in the hyper-technical world of the Medicare program, there must be adequate documentation in the medical record that the patient continues to suffer from disability of performing daily living activities following cataract surgery on the first eye. In the facts described above, the patient's statements about how well she can see following the first surgery could be the basis for a finding of no medical necessity for surgery on the second eye.

A technician examines a patient who complains of blurry vision and difficulty with reading and watching television. The patient articulates no other complaints in pursuing daily living activities. Upon examination, the patient appears to have a cataract and reflects a visual acuity of 20/30 under normal Snellen testing. To qualify for cataract surgery, the Medicare carrier requires a best-corrected visual acuity of 20/40 or worse under either Snellen or glare conditions. The technician then performs a brightness acuity test (BAT) with a glare level set on high. The patient "glares" to a visual acuity of 20/70, and the technician records it in the patient's chart as "20/70 with glare." The ophthalmologist confirms the findings of the technician, and the patient is determined to be a candidate for cataract surgery.

DOES THE PATIENT QUALIFY FOR CATARACT SURGERY UNDER MEDICARE REQUIREMENTS?

From the facts set forth above, it is not clear whether or not the patient would qualify for Medicare coverage. However, there are sufficient problems identified to suggest that there may be significant risk for the physician.

The Medicare statute requires that services must be reasonable and medically necessary. In order for cataract surgery to be medically necessary, three criteria must be met:

1. There must be the existence of a cataract.
2. The patient's visual acuity must meet prescribed objective criteria (in this case 20/40 or worse under either Snellen or glare conditions).
3. The patient must suffer from disability in pursuing daily living activities.

What is often overlooked, however, is that the objective criterion of visual acuity and the subjective criterion of disability in pursuing daily living activities must be linked. In this case, they are not. In the facts set forth above, the patient had no complaints about any glare-related disability. Yet, the patient's visual acuity without glare did not meet the objective visual acuity criterion to justify the medical necessity of the surgery. Instead, it was only when the BAT was used that the patient exhibited visual acuity of 20/40 or worse. If a patient articulates no glare-related disability, the Medicare program takes the position that a glare test cannot be used to justify surgery.

There also is an issue with respect to the operation of the glare test in this case. Futher operation of the BAT requires that the patient be first subjected to the low glare condition, followed by the medium glare condition. According to the package insert for the BAT, high glare is designed to simulate extraordinarily bright conditions, such as those experienced by airline pilots flying above the clouds. As a result, the Medicare program takes the position that high glare is not a basis to justify cataract surgery.

Finally, and closely related to the use of the BAT, the fact that the 20/70 visual acuity was recorded on the chart as "20/70 with glare" could be considered as misleading, as it does not indicate that the visual acuity was obtained as the result of a glare test at the high level which Medicare does not recognize. Practices must be careful to record accurately and completely all information related to diagnostic testing.

After attending a conference on fraud and abuse risk areas for ophthalmologists, the physicians of the Eye Treatment Institute (ETI) agree to implement a compliance program to ensure all ETI patients receive high-quality, medically necessary, and appropriately billed eye care services in compliance with all legal, regulatory, and ethical requirements. In order to identify potential billing and coding risks for ETI, their compliance attorney hires a consultant to audit a sample of ETI's medical and billing records. The consultant reports that of the 30 evaluation and management services (E/M) he reviewed, he disagreed with the level of code selected by the ETI physicians in 18 instances. According to the consultant, the documentation in the medical record did not support the level 4 or 5 E/M code selected in each instance. When the attorney and consultant meet with the ETI medical staff to discuss the documentation insufficiencies and methods to improve in this area, the physicians disagree with the consultant's findings, stating that regardless of the information found in the medical records, their patients are very complicated and, therefore, meet the CPT code requirements.

WHAT INFORMATION MUST A MEDICAL RECORD INCLUDE TO SUPPORT CLAIMS FOR E/M SERVICES?

The issue of proper coding is extremely complex, particularly in the area of E/M coding related to new and established patients. The CPT descriptor of the service represented by a particular code establishes the various components of care a physician must perform and document in order to bill for a particular service. Nevertheless, the medical community and government have long recognized the difficulties with the E/M codes and the documentation parameters used to justify billing a particular level code. In response, the Center for Medicare and Medicaid Services developed documentation guidelines (DGs) to supplement the CPT code descriptors. These guidelines specify what information must be in a patient's medical record in order to support billing at the various E/M levels.

The first DGs went into effect in September 1995 (1995 DGs) for use by carriers in performing medical review of E/M codes. The 1995 DGs drew immediate criticism because the documentation required to bill for a single system examination was not clear. It was felt that medical reviewers did not give credit for complete single-system physical examinations, and, therefore, it was impossible for specialists to meet the higher documentation requirements for the higher level E/M services. In response to this opposition, CMS developed a new set of guidelines, with assistance from the American Medical Association, that were intended to be more appropriate for single-system examinations (1997 DGs). The new guidelines were also intended to revise and clarify some of the information in the 1995 DGs.

The 1997 DGs require physicians to document a certain number of elements of a physical examination and assign numerical values to entries in the medical record. The level of E/M service is, in turn, intended to correlate to the "documentation score." The 1997 DGs were expected to replace the 1995 DGs; however, like the earlier version, physicians opposed the new guidelines on the basis that they were too complicated, too time consuming, and placed too much emphasis on documentation. In light of this opposition, CMS instructed carriers to use either the 1995 or 1997 DGs when reviewing medical records and committed to develop yet a third version of DGs. The third version, issued in draft in 1999, was to incorporate a multitude of clinical vignettes to help guide physicians' E/M code selections. But, once again, the DGs were criticized as creating a system that is too difficult to follow and could result in inconsistent review of providers.

To date, the 1999 DGs have not been finalized, and the Secretary of the Department of Health and Human Services testified before Congress that the clinical vignette project would be discontinued. Consequently, the 1995 and 1997 DGs stand as the relevant documentation guidance for physicians and other health care providers who submit claims for E/M services. While the ETI physicians may believe that the services rendered to their patients are consistent with certain E/M code descriptors, if the documentation in the relevant patient's medical record does not meet the documentation requirements outlined in either the 1995 or 1997 guidelines, the physicians are at significant risk for having payment for their services denied. Furthermore, ETI could face allegations of submitting false claims to the government if the physicians knowingly continue to submit claims for a level of service that is not reflected in the medical record. Without proper documentation, it is nearly impossible to prove that a service reflected on a claim form was the service actually received by the patient.

22

DOCUMENTATION REQUIREMENTS BEYOND MEDICARE

A 2-year-old child presents for an eye examination. Her mother is concerned that the child may need glasses, as she frequently squints. The child is uncooperative and the examination is difficult. The ophthalmologist makes minimal chart notes, and the chart is sent to the billing office to be filed as a comprehensive eye examination (code 92004).

Prior to submitting the claim to the third-party payor, the billing office reviews the chart notes and informs the physician that the documentation supports a level 1 E/M code (99201). The mother completed the registration form but ignored the history form. The exam notes state that the patient "fixates and follows," and that her pupil size appears normal. The physician writes, "deferred for intraocular pressure." There are no further chart notes. His assessment is normal eye exam.

The physician responds to his staff member that, *"This isn't Medicare, so I don't have to comply with all those rules."*

DO THE DOCUMENTATION GUIDELINES EXTEND BEYOND MEDICARE?

The basic principles of chart documentation extend beyond Medicare and apply to all types of medical and surgical services:

✧ The medical record should be complete and legible.

✧ Each encounter should include:

- Date of service
- Subjective complaint
- History relevant to the complaint
- Exam findings
- Assessment

- Plan
- Legible identity of provider (ie, signature)

The selection of the appropriate level of service is based on the documentation of these basic elements. The existence or type of third-party payor has no bearing when considering the need for these basic documentation requirements.

The patient's medical record validates the appropriateness of the services provided. Also, it is the basis for coding and billing by:

1. Verifying that the services were performed
2. Validating where they were performed
3. Describing the extent of services

Documented notations may vary when certain circumstances are present. An exam element may be considered performed if it is deferred because it is medically contraindicated, rather than overlooked or postponed due to patient preference. For example, dilation may be contraindicated if the patient presents with narrow anterior chamber angles. A notation is made to reflect the absence of dilation and the medical contraindication. Leaving an exam element blank means it was ignored and no credit is given.

The examination of a child, as referenced in the case study, is another example in which traditional documentation of the elements may not be possible. For example, the assessment of the anterior segment may be performed using a penlight if the child is unable to sit still behind the slit lamp. Chart notation for the anterior chamber and lens might read "grossly normal w/penlight." However, the absence of a notation means the element was not examined.

Documentation guidelines extend beyond Medicare, and the threat of a postpayment review exists with any payer. Furthermore, the need for thorough documentation extends beyond reimbursement. The medical record serves as a tool to treat the patient and as a means to communicate the patient's care to others.

Dr. A, a retina specialist, has a standing order in his practice that whenever fluorescein angiography (CPT 92235) is performed, fundus photography (CPT 92250) should be performed as well. Rather than wasting an entire roll of film for a few photos, the staff keeps the film in the camera until the roll is used. When the film is returned from the developer, the staff member labels the photos, places them in a plastic sheet, and files them in the respective patient's chart. Dr. A never reviews the fundus photos until the next patient visit, if then. No interpretation of the fundus photos is performed; only the fluorescein angioplasty was interpreted. Claims were filed as 92235 and 92250.

IS THE BILLING FOR BOTH THE FLUORESCEIN ANGIOGRAPHY AND FUNDUS PHOTO APPROPRIATE?

The definition in the CPT book for 92250 is fundus photography with interpretation and report. Interpretation and report means the physician must review the results and document his or her findings in the chart. The CPT book describes interpretation and report under the special ophthalmological services section as:

> Interpretation and report by the physician is an integral part of special ophthalmological services where indicated. Technical procedures (which may or may not be performed by the physician personally) are often part of the service, but should not be mistaken to constitute the service itself.

In the description above, the fundus photos were never reviewed, nor were findings documented. Therefore, Medicare and many other payors would only allow the technical component of this service; the professional component would be considered an overpayment. In some cases, the technical component may be denied as well, under the theory that without the interpretation, the service was of no value to the patient.

Additionally, no order was written in the patient's chart for the fundus photography, only for the fluorescein angiography. While standing orders may be accepted in certain settings, they raise concerns about the justification for the test. A question will almost certainly be raised concerning the medical necessity of a fundus photograph in every case where only medical necessity of the fluorescein angiography is documented. Even if the medical necessity could be established in all cases, failure to have a specific order in the record may risk a finding of lack of documentation.

24

Confirming Carrier Coding Advice

There is a difference of opinion within a large ophthalmic practice regarding a coding question, and the practice administrator brings the question to the compliance officer. The compliance officer believes that the practice codes the service appropriately, but he wants to be certain. Accordingly, the compliance officer contacts the carrier and asks the question. On the phone, the carrier representative confirms that the practice's current understanding of the coding criteria is correct. The compliance officer calls the practice administrator and tells him to continue as before, as the carrier has confirmed the practice's current use of the code.

Is Telephone Advice From the Carrier Adequate to Protect Practice?

At first glance, the administrator and the compliance officer have done everything correctly to protect the practice. Uncertain about a compliance issue, the practice contacted the carrier and confirmed the correct use. This should, one would expect, ensure that (1) the practice is acting on correct guidance, and (2) if the advice were incorrect, the practice's reliance on the carrier would protect it if enforcement authorities question the practice's policies or billings. Unfortunately, neither expectation is necessarily the case. Because carriers do not always interpret the Medicare requirements correctly or the same as the Center of Medicare and Medicaid Services (CMS), there is no guarantee that the carrier advice is correct. However, there are several ways a practice can minimize its exposure in such cases. The key is documentation. Appropriate documentation will help establish that the practice's reliance on the carrier advice was reasonable.

In its compliance guidance for physician practices, the Office of the Inspector General (OIG) recommends that physician practices document efforts to comply with applicable federal health care program requirements. The OIG suggests that practices document and retain records of requests and any written or oral responses. This step is extremely important if the practice intends to rely on the carrier response to guide it in future decisions, actions, or reimbursement requests. A written inquiry, with a written response, is preferred and should be obtained whenever possible.

If, for some reason, written confirmation is not possible, the practice should take steps to protect itself. The OIG has suggested that a practice maintain a log of oral inquiries between the practice and carrier representatives. The log should include the date of the call, the phone number called, the name (first and last) of the person at the carrier to whom the compliance officer or other personnel spoke, the question asked, and the answer, all as close to verbatim as possible. In addition, the practice should write a letter to the carrier, stating the oral advice received and the practice's intention to rely on the advice. The letter should request that the carrier advise the practice if the practice's understanding is incorrect. Such documentation should help protect the practice in the event that the carrier representative's oral advice turn out to be incorrect.

TOO MANY YAGS WITHIN
THE POSTOPERATIVE PERIOD

Dr. A is an extremely busy cataract surgeon who performs several thousand cataract surgeries per year. He also performs a large number of YAG capsulotomies. During a quality assurance review of these surgeries for the ambulatory surgery center (ASC), the reviewers noted that almost all of the YAGs were performed within 90 days of the initial cataract surgery.

WILL THE YAGS BE COVERED?

There are several concerns. In the Medicare population, most surgeons perform two to four YAG capsulotomies for every 10 cataract surgeries with intraocular lenses. Those YAG capsulotomies are usually performed within 12 to 36 months of the initial cataract surgery and are rarely required within the first 90 days postoperation. For a large volume of cataract surgeries, it is reasonable to expect a large number of YAG capsulotomies, but not so close to the primary cataract operation.

This elevated utilization makes the practice a target for scrutiny. On review, a Medicare auditor will apply the national policy (CIM §35 to 52) to determine the validity of a claim and the medical necessity for the procedure. The policy states that YAG capsulotomies within the 90-day postoperative period should be rare and uncommon within the first six months. When a YAG is performed within the global period, the payor requires additional chart documentation to support the medical necessity (ie, preoperative uveitis, chronic glaucoma, diabetes mellitus, prolonged use of pilocarpine, etc). The policy also addresses glare as an indication for YAG capsulotomy. Glare test results must show consensual light testing decreases visual acuity by two lines, or decrease in two lines of visual acuity in a glare tester. YAG capsulotomy should not be performed prophylactically or scheduled routinely at particular times after cataract surgery.

Unusual practice patterns merit special attention and oftentimes attract scrutiny from regulators. Dr. B should review his past cases, surgical indications, and the national Medicare payment policy. With that information, he should re-examine his protocol for YAG capsulotomy.

USING MEDICARE UTILIZATION DATA TO IDENTIFY POTENTIAL CODING ISSUES

A solo ophthalmologist practicing general ophthalmology struggled with the transition from use of ophthalmology CPT codes (920xx) to use of the evaluation and management (E/M) CPT codes (992xx). Without careful review of the criteria for the E/M codes, the physician began to file claims, generally applying CPT codes 99214 and 99215.

The Medicare carrier selected the physician for a comprehensive medical review due to a significant variance between his practice patterns and that of his peers. The carrier review determined that the documentation did not support the level of care billed for several of the claims in the sample. The carrier issued an overpayment determination relating to the E/M codes used during the period in question.

HOW COULD THE PHYSICIAN IDENTIFY THE POTENTIAL PROBLEM BEFORE MEDICARE IDENTIFIED IT?

Utilization profiles are a useful tool to Medicare carriers as an indicator of potential problems. Physicians can use similar information to predict areas of potential scrutiny by comparing their practice patterns with national norms. Physicians should recognize that using such data is not foolproof, as practice patterns throughout the United States are not uniform and there may be special circumstances that support extraordinary utilization rates. As always, the chart documentation must support the service. Nevertheless, these data can serve to identify potential problems early.

In the case study, it would have been useful if the physician knew that his utilization of high-level exams was disproportionate to Medicare's expected utilization. Special circumstances did not exist to support the extraordinary rates. The 2000 Part B Extract and Summary System data for the codes in question provide a frame of reference:

- ✧ Nine of every 100 established patient exams filed by ophthalmologists were filed with 99214.
- ✧ One of every 100 established patient exams filed by ophthalmologists were filed with 99215.
- ✧ Thirty-three of every 100 established patient exams filed by ophthalmologists were filed with 92014.

Beyond the utilization data, the physician should have paid close attention to the stricter documentation guidelines associated with 99214 and 99215 as compared to the ophthalmology codes (920xx).

In 1997, the Center of Medicare and Medicaid Services (CMS) released documentation guidelines for single-system specialty examinations utilizing E/M codes. E/M code documentation has three components: history, examination, and medical decision-making. The 1997 guidelines provide specific criteria for the ocular examination. The history and decision-making components are consistent for all specialties. The higher-level E/M codes (992x4 and 992x5) require extensive documentation for these three components.

While CMS has not published a national policy for the ophthalmology CPT codes (920xx), many Medicare carriers publish *General Ophthalmological Services* local policies. There are, however, differences among the policies. In the absence of published guidelines by a carrier, the CPT handbook provides documentation requirements.

Overutilization of Punctal Occlusion With Plugs

After reading a variety of articles discussing punctal occlusion with plugs and listening to a manufacturer's representative as well as other ophthalmologists, Dr. A began offering this service to her patients. Dry eye symptoms and the benefits of punctal occlusion with plugs were described in literature throughout the office as well as the "message-on-hold" recording on the practice's telephone system. The technicians and office staff were trained to ask patients about symptoms related to dry eye and to provide patients with brochures discussing the procedure. Dr. A adopted an aggressive treatment protocol that includes insertion of collagen plugs in all four puncta, followed by silicone plugs in the lower puncta 10 to 14 days later. Silicone plugs in the upper puncta were used as a third step only when the first two silicone plugs did not provide symptomatic relief.

In the first 3 months of providing this service, Dr. A performs punctal occlusion on 21% of her patients. The majority of these patients had the procedure with both the collagen and silicone plugs.

Does This Clinical Protocol Cause Concern?

Increasing utilization of punctual occlusion with plugs over the past few years has drawn attention from payors that may result in overpayment determinations. A little extra caution is warranted whenever there is rapid growth in any new procedure. In particular, it is important to document the patient's complaint(s), history of the present illness, indications for the procedure, objective findings of the exam, results of diagnostic tests for dry eye, and the manner in which the punctal occlusion was performed (ie, which punctum, kind of plug, etc).

Under Medicare regulations, reimbursement is made only for medically necessary procedures. Punctal occlusion is not medically necessary for every patient who presents with symptoms of dry eye syndrome. Furthermore, the standard of care for the treatment of dry eye is to begin with artificial tears and lubricating ointments before a more invasive therapy such as punctal occlusion. According to American Academy of Ophthalmology treatment guidelines, when occlusion is necessary, the vast majority of patients with moderate dry eye require occlusion only of the lower puncta. Occlusion of the upper puncta is required only when severe disease is present or for those patients who do not obtain symptomatic relief following the occlusion of the lower puncta.

Aging of the population and the popularity of laser-assisted in situ keratomileusis, commonly known as LASIK, have resulted in an increasing number of patients needing treatment for dry eye. These factors, combined with the higher reimbursement for the procedure, have transformed punctal occlusion into a very popular procedure. For this reason, physicians must pay extra attention to chart notes, claims for reimbursement, and the medical protocol for utilizing this procedure.

28

MARKETING

An ophthalmologist has hired an advertising agency to assist in promoting her practice. The advertising agency develops a comprehensive ad campaign and presents it to the ophthalmologist for review and approval. The advertising promotes the ophthalmologist as being "one of the best surgeons in the area," describes her surgery technique as "painless," and "guarantees that the surgery will improve your eyesight." In addition, the ad contains a quote from one of the practice's happy patients saying that "one day after my refractive surgery, I was 20/20 and had no problems."

IS THE AD COPY ACCEPTABLE?

The advertisement described above contains a number of serious problems. Both the Federal Trade Commission (FTC), as well as several state medical boards, have taken action against physicians whose advertising is considered to be false or misleading. Any advertising to the public must be truthful, and all facts stated must be capable of being substantiated. Further, any description of results must reflect the results of the typical patient. Some states have even more restrictive provisions, such as a prohibition on claims of superiority or the use of patient testimonials.

With respect to the advertisement in question, while it may be a true statement that the physician is one of the best surgeons in the area, that is a claim that is very hard to substantiate. Furthermore, in a state that prohibits claims of superiority, even if the statement could be substantiated, it may be prohibited. The suggestion that surgery is "painless" is always a red flag. The use of anesthetic or the need to prescribe even over-the-counter painkillers for postsurgery treatment is an acknowledgement that this surgery is not painless. "Painless" is a word to avoid in any marketing. The "guarantee that the surgery will improve your eyesight" is also problematic, as there is no assurance that this will be true in every case. Finally, the use of the patient testimonial is also likely to be a problem without some type of qualifier that results may vary from patient-to-patient. As indicated above, some states prohibit the use of any patient testimonials. While the constitutionality of such prohibition is subject to challenge, any such challenge will be expensive and time consuming. If a physician is in a state that prohibits patient testimonials, he or she should consider the potential risk carefully before using them in marketing.

29

INFORMED CONSENT

A patient arrives 15 minutes late for her appointment at her physician's office for an office-based surgery. Upon checking in with the receptionist, she is handed several informed consent forms and is told to "hurry up and fill these out." The patient is then told that if she has any questions, a nurse is available to answer or assist, and is instructed to take a seat in the waiting area. The patient signs the forms, returns them to the receptionist, and does not ask to speak with a nurse.

HAS THE PATIENT GIVEN INFORMED CONSENT?

Many physicians believe that so long as a patient has signed the informed consent form, the physician has fulfilled the "informed consent" requirement and is protected. A signed piece of paper, however, is not a guarantee of informed consent. Rather, informed consent is a process designed to ensure that a patient understands the risks and benefits of various medical procedures, as well as the alternatives to that treatment, and, absent physician negligence, to protect physicians from liability for those risks that the patient assumes. Although a signed informed consent form is strong evidence of the patient's awareness, it is not uncommon for courts to look past the document itself and determine if true informed consent took place.

A complete informed consent process should:
1. Describe the procedure for which the patient is being asked to give consen
2. Discuss the attendant risks and benefits
3. Notify the patient of alternative courses of treatment in a way in which the patient understands the information

4. Provide the patient with sufficient time to process the information

5. Provide meaningful opportunity for questions.

There are several informed consent issues raised in the described scenario. First, patients must be given sufficient time to digest the information that has been provided to them. In the above scenario, although it is not the physician's fault that the patient arrived late for her appointment, a rushed signature on a consent form is unlikely to provide time for the patient to read and understand the information.

Second, patients should be given a meaningful opportunity to ask questions of their physician about the information presented. In the described scenario, the patient clearly did not have a meaningful opportunity to ask questions. In part, this was due to the rushed nature of this particular encounter. Even under these circumstances, however, when the patient was taken to the office for the procedure, a nurse should have reviewed the informed consent form with the patient, making certain that the patient had, in fact, reviewed and understood it, and encouraged the patient to ask questions if necessary.

Finally, beyond having a nurse review the form with the patient, ultimately, it is the physician who performs the procedure and who is responsible for obtaining a patient's informed consent. It is the operating physician's duty as well as in his or her best interest to assure a patient has made an informed decision as to whether to submit to a proposed procedure. The best way for a physician to ensure and be confident that the patient understands the information is to participate personally in the process and be available for questions.

30

Use of Scribes to Complete a Superbill

A large ophthalmology practice uses a scribe system to speed the documentation process and improve patient flow. It is the policy of the practice for scribes to fill out the history and physical examination form, the progress notes, and the charge form, including entering the ICD-9 and CPT codes. During an audit of the practice's documentation system, the compliance officer discovered that many of the physicians sign the scribe's notes and the charge form without verifying that the content of the forms is correct. At the next medical staff meeting, the compliance officer advises the physicians that they must review the information in the medical record and on the charge form for accuracy before affixing their signature because the government will hold them accountable for the content. The physicians argue that it is the scribe's responsibility to ensure the information is correct, not theirs.

Who is Correct: The Physicians or the Compliance Officer?

The compliance officer. The documentation in a patient's medical record and on a charge form is a confirmation of the physician's decision regarding the services ordered, the services performed, and the clinical basis for ordering those services. In its Compliance Program Guidance for Individual and Small Group Physician Practices, the Office of the Inspector General (OIG) made clear that health care providers have a duty to reasonably ensure that claims submitted for their services to any federally funded health care programs are true and accurate (65 Fed. Reg. 59434-Oct. 5, 2000). The OIG also explained that the CPT and ICD-9 codes reported on health insurance claims forms must be supported by the medical record, and that the record should contain all necessary information to validate including:

1. Site of service
2. Appropriateness of the services provided

3. Accuracy of the billing

4. Identity of the caregiver

In a situation where a scribe fails to select the appropriate procedure or diagnosis codes or fails to document services correctly, such as under the facts described above, the government could take the position that the practice physicians acted recklessly within the meaning of the federal Civil False Claims Act by delegating his or her responsibility for documentation and coding to nonclinicians and not reviewing the scribe's decisions. In order for the practice to manage its risk under the False Claims Act, the physicians either must complete all documentation, or at a minimum, the physicians must review the scribe's medical record entries and code selections to ensure they are correct.

31

INFORMED CONSENT AND OFF-LABEL USE

FACTS

A physician uses a laser in refractive surgery. The laser has been approved by the FDA for use up to 12 diopters. A patient presents with a refractive error of -14. The physician examines the patient and concludes that he is a good candidate for surgery. The patient is provided with an informed consent form describing the risks, benefits, and alternatives to surgery. In neither the informed consent form, nor in the discussion with the physician, is the patient advised of the off-label use of the laser.

DOES OFF-LABEL USE REQUIRE A DIFFERENT INFORMED CONSENT?

There is no legal restriction against a physician employing a laser for an off-label use. Physicians are recognized as having the right to exercise their professional medical judgment within the scope of their practice. Because such off-label use has become commonplace, in such cases patients frequently are given no additional information about off-label use. From a risk management perspective, however, it is always safer to assure that the patient is fully informed about all of the elements involved in a particular procedure, including the fact that the physician intends to employ a laser for an off-label use.

This issue is one that is rarely tested. The adequacy of the informed consent becomes an issue only in the context of malpractice litigation. If there is a bad result, however, a plaintiff's attorney will almost certainly focus on the adequacy of the informed consent. Failure to include information relating to off-label use will be an attractive argument to make to the jury. It is an argument that can be minimized significantly if the patient has received the information as part of the informed consent process.

LEGAL ISSUES

32

COMANAGEMENT CONTRACTS

An ophthalmologist is approached by an optometrist with a very large patient base. The optometrist proposes that they enter into a formal comanagement relationship where the optometrist will agree to refer all of his cataract and refractive surgery patients to the ophthalmologist if the ophthalmologist agrees to refer all of those patients back to the optometrist for postoperative care. Under the arrangement, the ophthalmologist will collect all of the fees for the services rendered and will pay the optometrist for the optometrist's services. They agree that the optometrist will be paid 20% of the surgical fee in the case of cataract surgery, and 40% of the surgical fee for refractive procedures. In order to be certain that there is no misunderstanding, they decide to put their agreements in writing.

IS A FORMAL COMANAGEMENT AGREEMENT BETWEEN AN OPHTHALMOLOGIST AND OPTOMETRIST APPROPRIATE?

The proposed arrangement has several problems. As a general matter, there never should be an agreement between an ophthalmologist and an optometrist to refer patients to each other, whether that agreement is written or oral. Comanagement must be determined to be in the patient's best interest and, most importantly, must be undertaken only when the patient chooses to participate in a comanagement arrangement.

The "terms" of the proposed agreement reflect problems as well. With respect to Medicare patients, if the optometrist performs a service, the optometrist must bill for the service. Medicare reassignment rules prohibit the ophthalmologist from billing for services performed by an optometrist in another practice. The 80%-20% split for surgery versus postoperative care reflects the Medicare prescribed amount, presuming the optometrist performs postoperative care for the full 90-day period.

The 60%-40% split for refractive surgery may or may not present a problem. The obvious question presented is whether the amount received by the optometrist reflects the fair market value of services performed by the optometrist. If the answer is yes, then the arrangement is defensible. If not, the strong suggestion will be that the amount above the fair market value reflects a payment for the referral.

Both ophthalmologists and optometrists must be very cautious in connection with comanagement relationships relating to refractive surgery. There is frequently a belief that because such services are not paid for by Medicare or Medicaid, the traditional fraud and abuse analysis does not apply. This view is incorrect. Many states have anti-kickback laws that are similar to the federal law, and those that do not have specific anti-kickback laws are likely to have provisions in the state licensing acts that are sufficiently broad to prohibit conduct that could be characterized as a kickback. In this case, however, even if there is no state anti-kickback law at issue, the optometrist had agreed to refer cataract surgery cases covered by Medicare. This could cause the federal Anti-Kickback Statute to be triggered as the result of a higher than appropriate payment for the optometrist in connection with the refractive surgery referrals.

COMANAGEMENT SERVICES
COVERED BY COMMERCIAL INSURANCE

A patient covered by commercial insurance is diagnosed with cataracts. The patient meets the insurer's criteria for coverage of the surgery. The patient has advised the ophthalmologist that he understands that his optometrist is licensed to provide postoperative services and that he wishes to return to his optometrist for the provision of postoperative services. The commercial insurer, however, does not recognize optometrists as part of its physician panel.

The ophthalmologist is familiar with the optometrist's abilities and, where appropriate, has successfully comanaged other cataract surgery patients with the optometrist. In order to accommodate the patient, the ophthalmologist bills the commercial insurer, is paid a global fee for the cataract surgery and postoperative care, and pays the optometrist an amount for the postoperative services consistent with the Medicare reimbursement guidelines. The ophthalmologist provided the appropriate educational statement and informed consent to the patient just as he does for Medicare patients whenever he comanages cataract surgery. The patient confirmed his understanding about the need for postoperative services, the difference between an ophthalmologist and an optometrist, and his choice to obtain postoperative care from the optometrist.

MAY THE OPHTHALMOLOGIST COLLECT
THE GLOBAL FEE AND PAY THE OPTOMETRIST?

While the end result of this arrangement is identical with the legally supportable comanagement relationship involving Medicare patients, there are a number of issues that are triggered. First, many states prohibit physicians from splitting part of their professional fee with another practitioner outside the practice, even if it is in return for the provision of professional services. It is important, therefore, to review the law in the state in which this arrangement is proposed.

Second, the provider agreement between the ophthalmologist and the commercial insurer, or the policies developed by the commercial insurer, may similarly prohibit sharing of fees with any practitioner who is not included in the physician panel. Therefore, even if there is no state law prohibition, such an arrangement may violate the terms of the agreement between the ophthalmologist and the insurer, and may threaten termination of the ophthalmologist's participation on that insurer's panel.

Generally, however, there will be no clear guidance either in state law or in the provider agreement or policies issued by the commercial insurer. In order to avoid potential liability, the ophthalmologist should send a letter to the insurer and advise that one of the insurer's subscribers has expressed an interest in obtaining services by an optometrist licensed to perform such services. The ophthalmologist should either seek approval of the proposal, or, at a minimum, advise the insurer that the ophthalmologist intends to follow the Medicare guidelines in compensating the optometrist for the services provided, unless the insurer advises the ophthalmologist that such an arrangement is inappropriate. If the insurer objects, the ophthalmologist should explain to the patient that it is the insurer that is preventing the proposed arrangement from going forward.

A similar inquiry to the state Board of Medicine may also be appropriate and is strongly recommended in those states where the fee split laws appear to prohibit such an arrangement.

34

LEASE OF SPACE FROM AN OPTOMETRIST

An ophthalmologist receives referrals from an optometrist in another part of the state. The patient flow becomes significant enough that the ophthalmologist decides that, for the convenience of these patients, he will open a satellite office that he will visit periodically, at least 1 day per month. The most logical location is the office of the optometrist, who has a suite of offices that are not always busy.

The parties sign a lease agreement with the following terms:

1. The ophthalmologist will lease "a lane" from the optometry practice.
2. The ophthalmologist will have use of the lane 1 day per month, or as the parties may otherwise determine from time-to-time.
3. The rental fee will be $X per each patient seen by the ophthalmologist in the rented space.

The parties did not engage a consultant or otherwise perform an analysis of the fair market value of the space.

DOES THE LEASE BETWEEN OPHTHALMOLOGIST AND OPTOMETRIST PRESENT ANY PROBLEMS?

Any lease between an ophthalmologist and an optometrist who refers patients to that ophthalmologist will raise questions concerning whether the terms of the lease violate the Anti-Kickback Statute. In fact, in February 2000, the Office of the Inspector General (OIG) published a special *Fraud Alert* on the rental of space in physician offices by persons or entities to which the physicians refer.

The *Fraud Alert* identified practices that the OIG believes are "questionable features" of space leases. Among the questionable features identified by the OIG are the rental fees that vary with the number of patients (or referrals). The lease in the described scenario includes such a provision. Because the rental fee varies based on the number of patients seen, the clear incentive for the landlord/optometrist is to refer patients to the ophthalmologist. The OIG would find this to be problematic.

Second, from the facts presented, there is no assurance that the parties established a rental fee that reflects fair market value. An ability to demonstrate the fair market value of the space is crucial to any defense against accusations of impropriety. Another concern relates to the potential variability of the terms of the agreement. Instead of establishing a fixed frequency for the use of the space by the ophthalmologist, in this scenario the physician's use may vary, presumably depending on the volume of patients to be seen.

Fortunately, however, there is a *safe harbor* to the federal statute that protects lease arrangements meeting certain requirements. The space lease safe harbor requires that there be a written agreement for at least a 1-year term, and that the agreement covers all of the premises leased between the parties. Further, the aggregate rental charge under the agreement must be set in advance, reflect fair market value for the space, and may not vary with the volume or value of referrals between the parties. The safe harbor also requires that the aggregate space leased may not exceed a commercially reasonable amount given the business purpose of the agreement. Finally, if the lease is part-time, the agreement must specify exactly the schedule or intervals and state the exact rent for such intervals.

At first glance, the safe harbor requirements may appear burdensome. However, the high-profile relationship between optometrists and ophthalmologists makes remunerative agreements between them likely targets for government enforcement action. Combined with the relative ease with which space leases can meet the safe harbor requirements, parties to such arrangements should make every effort to do so, as the benefit of fitting within a safe harbor is significant.

BILLING ISSUES RELATING TO LASIK

An ophthalmologist performs laser-assisted in situ keratomileusis (LASIK) at a laser center owned and operated by an independent third party. Many of the ophthalmologist's patients are referred by local optometrists with whom the patients have long-standing relationships. An optometrist advises his patients about the availability of the procedure, which has a global fee for the surgery of $2000 per eye. The optometrist then explains to the patient about the need for postoperative care, which he can perform if the patient chooses. The patient agrees to have the procedure and states that he wishes to return to the optometrist for postoperative care.

At the center, the patient is educated further about postoperative care options and confirms his decision to return to his optometrist. The patient is then instructed to make the payment in the name of the center. The center assures the patient that it will take care of making payments to the surgeon and optometrist. In fact, of the $2000 fee per eye, the center keeps $1000, $500 is paid to the surgeon, and the remaining $500 is paid to the comanaging optometrist. This information, however, is not disclosed to the patient at any time.

MUST THE PATIENT BE INFORMED
ABOUT THE DIVISION OF THE GLOBAL FEE?

While the facts set forth above assume that the patient has been properly educated about the need for postoperative care and has made a voluntary informed choice to return to the optometrist for the provision of postoperative care, there is still a problem with the arrangement. Specifically, the patient has not been informed which portion of the payment goes to each party for the provision of services. Although there is no requirement similar to the Medicare program rule that each provider must bill for the services he or she performs, the patient should be advised how much he or she is paying for the components of the surgery. Therefore, if the vision center serves as the "collection agent" for itself, the ophthalmologist, and the optometrist, there should be an itemized statement on the bill to reflect the amount to be paid to each of the three parties. In this way, the patient is able to make an informed choice about whether he or she believes that $500 per eye is an appropriate payment for the postoperative services.

This scenario also raises the question of whether the amount paid to the optometrist is consistent with fair market value for the services performed. If the amount is grossly in excess of what would be considered fair market value for the services performed, there is the risk of a kickback allegation in those states that have anti-kickback laws. While the risk of such an allegation is reduced if there is full disclosure to the patient, fair market value for the postoperative care must always be a consideration in any comanagement relationship.

36

OPTOMETRIST-CONTROLLED REFRACTIVE CENTER

A group of optometrists decides to establish a refractive surgery center. The optometrists raise the necessary capital, lease space and equipment, and hire technicians and other staff necessary for the operation of the center. Assume for the purposes of this discussion that there are no state licensing or certificate of need laws that apply.

The optometrists identify an ophthalmologist who is a skilled surgeon and interested in avoiding the administrative hassles of operating a practice. The ophthalmologist agrees to perform surgery at the refractive center, and agrees to the terms proposed by the optometrists. Specifically, the refractive center will charge $2000 per eye, $500 of which will go to the surgeon, $500 of which will go to the optometrist performing the postoperative care, and $1000 will go to the center. In addition, while not part of the arrangement, the optometrists now refer all of their cataract surgery patients to the same ophthalmologist, who performs that surgery at the local hospital. Previously, the optometrists had referred their cataract surgery to several different ophthalmologists in town.

IS THE ARRANGEMENT BETWEEN THE OPTOMETRISTS AND THE OPHTHALMOLOGIST ACCEPTABLE?

Reference is made to the scenarios describing comanagement and billing issues relating to LASIK. The legal issues described in those scenarios apply equally to the fact pattern above. Additional issues, however, are raised here. First, certain states prohibit the corporate practice of medicine and apply that restriction fairly rigorously. There is a risk that the corporate practice of medicine prohibition could be triggered to the extent that the facts create the appearance that either the laser center or the optometrists dictate how the surgeon performs services. Generally, however, this problem is avoided as long as there is no interference by the optometrists or the refractive center in the ophthalmologist's performance of services.

Second, several states impose a restriction against physicians splitting fees with nonphysicians or others outside of the physician's practice. Here, again, as long as the parties follow the billing rules set forth in Chapter 35, the fee-split issue should be avoided.

Most importantly, however, this scenario identifies a potential problem with respect to the change in optometrists' referral pattern for cataract surgery patients. While not a violation per se, such a transfer in referral pattern will undoubtedly raise red flags. The refractive surgery arrangement with the optometrists could trigger an inquiry as to whether the ophthalmologist is providing the optometrists with something of value, and in return, receiving referrals for cataract surgery covered by Medicare. If the government believes that the change in referral pattern was, in fact, the result of the provision of something of value (such as an unreasonably high comanagement fee or the willingness to accept a reduced surgery fee, thereby allowing the optometrists to retain a high laser center fee), there is the risk of an allegation that the federal Anti-Kickback Statute has been violated. Such an allegation must be supported by evidence that the parties knowingly and willfully intended to enter into such an arrangement. Because the government would be required to develop such evidence by testimony about the initial discussion between the parties in setting up the arrangement, it is critical that no suggestion be made that any benefit is provided to the optometrists and that all of the arrangements reflect arms' length, fair market value agreements.

INVESTMENT IN AN AMBULATORY SURGERY CENTER

An ophthalmic surgeon has been offered an opportunity to buy into a local, multispecialty ambulatory surgery center (ASC). She is offered shares equal to a 10% ownership interest in the ASC. The per-share price is 25% less than the per-share price offered to a surgeon investor last year. The surgeon will receive profit distributions consistent with her 10% ownership interest. Further, the shareholder agreement states that there is no requirement that the surgeon perform her surgical procedures at the ASC. The ASC typically offers to loan all or part of the purchase price to an investing surgeon, at 6% interest.

DOES THE PROPOSED INVESTMENT IN THE ASC CONSTITUTE A KICKBACK VIOLATION?

The principal issue implicated by this scenario is the federal Anti-Kickback Statute. The Anti-Kickback Statute makes it a criminal offense to knowingly offer or receive remuneration in return for the referral of an individual for the purpose of supplying items or services that may be covered by a federal health care program. *Remuneration* includes anything of value, given directly or indirectly, overtly or covertly, in cash or in kind. In the above scenario, the surgeon is in a position to refer procedures to the ASC and will receive items of value from the ASC in the form of profit distributions, reduced per share price, and a loan on advantageous terms.

The question, then, is whether the physician's ownership interest would qualify for a *safe harbor* to the federal statute. Because of the broad language of the statute, which could encompass legitimate arrangements that do not present the potential for abuse, Congress authorized the development of regulations, known as safe harbors, which provide protection for certain conduct that would otherwise violate the statute. Safe harbors have specific requirements, and an arrangement not meeting the requirements exactly will fall outside the protection of the safe harbor. Failure to meet a safe harbor, however, does not necessarily mean that an arrangement is illegal.

There is a particular safe harbor that protects investments in four different types of ASCs. The OIG's overriding theme with the ASC safe harbor is that the ASC should function as an extension of the investing physician's practice. Within that context, there are many complicated requirements, only some of which are discussed below. In particular, there is a safe harbor for ownership in multi-specialty ASCs.

The ASC interests in the above scenario would not meet an ASC safe harbor for a variety of reasons. First, one of the safe harbor conditions is that loans to a potential investor from the entity or other investors for the purpose of investing are prohibited. Thus, the parties in the above scenario should be aware that if the ASC makes a loan to an investing surgeon, the ASC would no longer fit the safe harbor. Once outside the safe harbor, the loan terms would be examined by the OIG for a determination of whether the terms, such as the low interest rate, are fair market values.

In addition, the reduced per-share sale price for this particular investor might remove the arrangement from the protection of ASC safe harbor. This is because the amount paid to an investor in return for the investment must be directly proportional to the amount of the investor's capital investment. Although at first glance, a profit distribution proportional to the ownership interest would meet this requirement, the reduced per-share price would raise the question as to whether the investing surgeon's return is proportional to his capital investment. Failing to meet the safe harbor on this particular issue could be risky because the OIG would be very concerned about the receipt by the surgeon of his shares for less than fair market value and might view the reduced price to be remuneration in exchange for referrals. This concern could be mitigated, however, if the parties received an independent fair market valuation of the shares before purchase.

As a further condition, one of the relevant ASC safe harbor requirements is that an investing physician who refers procedures to the ASC must derive at least one-third of his or her medical practice income from his or her own performance of surgical procedures that are on the Medicare-approved ASC procedure list. Note that this criterion does not require that all of the procedures be performed in the ASC; instead it merely requires that the income be derived from the surgical procedures on the ASC list.

Finally, because the ASC is multispecialty, there is an additional requirement for the physician investors. Specifically, at least one-third of the surgical procedures performed by each physician investor must be performed at the particular ASC in which he or she is investing.

Although a failure to meet the requirements of a safe harbor does not mean that a given arrangement is illegal, the fewer safe harbor requirements that an arrangement meets, the greater the chances of the OIG asserting that the arrangement is abusive.

Quality Eye Care, PC (QEC) and Outstanding Ophthalmology, PC (OO) both want to own and operate an optical shop to enhance the profitability of their group practices. The physicians in both groups realize, however, that their geographic area will not sustain two optical shops. As a result, the groups decide to enter into a joint venture to own and operate one optical shop, called Clear Vision, Inc (CV). The terms of the joint venture call for the ophthalmologists of both practices to own equal shares of CV, and for profits to be divided according to referrals to the optical shop. Both practices include Medicare patients, some of whom will obtain postcataract surgery eyeglasses from CV. Net profits related to business generated from other sources will be divided equally among all the physician-owners.

Does the Proposed Joint Venture Pose Any Legal Risk for the Physician-Owners?

Yes. Historically, ophthalmologists and optometrists were advised, and appropriately so, to refrain from entering into any type of investment or compensation arrangement involving an optical shop that was not part of his or her own practice or group practice. Such relationships ran afoul of the federal Physician Anti-Self-Referral Statute (or as it is commonly referred, the Stark Law). The Stark Law prohibits a physician from ordering a service that is provided by an entity that the physician or an immediate family member has a financial relationship if the service falls within one of the categories of designated health services (DHS) covered by the Stark Law, is reimbursed by Medicare or Medicaid, and if the financial relationship does not qualify for an exception. Until the release of the final Stark II regulations by the Center for Medicare and Medicaid Services (CMS) in January 2001, postcataract spectacles and lenses were considered part of the DHS category of prosthetic devices. Consequently, unless an optical shop arrangement fell within one of the Stark Law exceptions, referrals for post-cataract spectacles or lenses by a physician to an optical shop with which he or she had an investment or compensation relationship violated the Stark Law.

As of 2001, however, this limitation on physician ownership of optical shops was eliminated under the federal law as the result of regulations issued by CMS, which removed post-cataract spectacles and lenses from the list of DHS. Now, assuming an optical shop does not provide any other service that is considered a DHS, the Stark Law is not applicable to ventures involving optical shops.

Despite the elimination of the legal concerns raised by the Stark Law, optical shop joint ventures involving physicians who are both investors in the joint venture and who are in a position to refer to the joint venture may raise concern under the federal Anti-Kickback Statute. To the extent that ophthalmologists may profit from referrals of patients to optical shops in which the ophthalmologists have a financial interest, the federal Anti-Kickback Statute may be triggered.

The federal Anti-Kickback Statute prohibits the offer, solicitation, payment, or receipt of anything of value (direct or indirect, overt or covert, in cash or in kind) that is intended to induce the referral of a patient for an item or service that is reimbursed by a federal health care program, including Medicare or Medicaid. The law imposes liability to both sides of an impermissible "kickback" transaction and has been interpreted broadly by several courts to apply to situations where only one purpose of a payment is to induce referrals, notwithstanding the fact that there may be other legitimate purposes for which the payment is made. As a result, virtually any financial relationship in which a health care provider is a referral source, as is the case here, has potential anti-kickback implications.

Because the Anti-Kickback Statute, as drafted, would prohibit many practical and nonabusive ways of delivering health care, Congress adopted several exceptions to the law and granted the Office of the Inspector General (OIG) of the Department of Health and Human Services authority to except additional arrangements from the reach of the law through regulations called safe harbors. These safe harbors define practices that are not subject to the Anti-Kickback Statute because they are viewed by the government as being unlikely to result in fraud and abuse. Unfortunately, because of the narrow manner in which the safe harbor regulations are drafted, the existing safe harbors offer no protection under the presented facts. Failure to fit within a safe harbor, however, does not mean that an arrangement is illegal per se. Therefore, one must look to other guidance to determine the degree of risk involved.

One source of information is a publication by the OIG known as a *Fraud Alert*. Fraud Alerts are statements of the OIG's view on certain common arrangements. In 1989, the OIG issued a special *Fraud Alert on Joint Venture Arrangements under the Anti-Kickback Statute* (Special Fraud Alert) discussing joint venture arrangements that may violate the federal Anti-Kickback Statute. Though 12 years old, the document still remains useful for identifying factors of various investment structures that may increase or decrease liability under the Anti-Kickback Statute. The Special Fraud Alert identified three principal areas that the OIG would review when analyzing joint ventures: (1) the manner in which investors are selected, (2) the nature of the business structure of the arrangement, and (3) the financing and profit distributions. Specifically, the Special Fraud Alert identified the following "red flags" as indicators of potentially unlawful activity:

- Investors are chosen because they are in a position to make referrals.
- Physicians who are expected to make a large number of referrals may be offered a greater investment opportunity in the joint venture than those anticipated to make fewer referrals.
- Physician investors may be actively encouraged to make referrals to the joint venture and may be encouraged to divest their ownership interest if they fail to sustain an acceptable level of referrals.
- The joint venture tracks its sources of referrals and distributes this information to the investors.
- Investors may be required to divest their ownership interest if they cease to practice in the service area (eg, if they move, become disabled, or retire).

- Investment interests are nontransferable.

- The structure of the joint venture may be suspect, such as in the case of a *shell entity*. A shell entity is identified as one where there is very little capital, equipment, or other hard assets in the venture and another entity is responsible for the day-to-day operations of the joint venture.

- The amount of capital invested by the physician is disproportionately small and the return disproportionately large compared to a typical investment in a new business.

- Physician investors only invest a nominal amount, such as $500 to $1500.

- Investors are permitted to borrow the amount of the investment from the entity and pay it back through deductions from profit distributions.

- Investors may be paid extraordinary returns on the investment in comparison to the risks involved, often well over 50% to 100% per year.

While the optical shop venture likely avoids many of the concerns set forth in the Special Fraud Alert, there is one issue that should be addressed. In particular, the investors should not receive distributions based on the volume of their referrals to the business, but rather based solely on their equity ownership in CV. Other ways to reduce risk include extending the investment opportunity to non-referral sources.

39

A general ophthalmology practice contracts with a retina specialist to provide services to its patients. The agreement with the retina specialist is on a part-time basis and classifies the specialist as an independent contractor. The practice bills and receives payment for the office-based services provided by the retina specialist. The practice also bills and receives payment for surgical procedures provided to the practice's patients by the specialist at a nearby ambulatory surgery center. The practice's cataract surgeons and other nonophthalmology surgeons own the ambulatory surgery center. The retina specialist is paid 30% of the net collections attributable to the services he performs.

MAY THE PRACTICE BILL AND COMPENSATE A PHYSICIAN INDEPENDENT CONTRACTOR BASED ON A PERCENTAGE OF REVENUE GENERATED BY THE PHYSICIAN?

The proposed arrangement is not in compliance with the Medicare reassignment rules. Those rules generally prohibit anyone other than the person who actually provides a service from collecting the payment. There are exceptions to the reassignment prohibition; the most relevant allows a practice to bill for services rendered by an independent contractor, as long as those services are provided in premises owned or leased by the practice. While this would allow the practice to bill for the office-based services rendered by the specialist, since the ambulatory surgical center (ASC) is not an asset nor a wholly owned subsidiary of the practice, the practice may not bill for the surgery performed by the specialist at the ASC.

This arrangement also raises issues under the federal Anti-Kickback Statute as well as anti-kickback statutes in states that have similar prohibitions. The federal statute makes it a violation of both criminal and civil law for any person to knowingly and willfully pay anything, directly or indirectly, in cash or in kind, to reward or induce a referral for any service covered by a federally funded health care program. Safe harbor regulations promulgated by the Office of the Inspector General provide protection for certain personal service arrangements. To qualify for the safe harbor, however, payment must be fixed, set in advance, and not vary with the value or volume of referrals.

An arrangement need not comply with a safe harbor to avoid violating the statute, however. In situations where a safe harbor does not apply, the government is likely to focus on the question of whether a relationship reflects fair market value. Where it does not, there is concern that there may be intent to reward or induce referrals. Here, the government might question whether 30% reflects fair market value for the retina specialist's services, or, perhaps more appropriately, since the practice is the source of referrals for the retina specialist, whether the practice's retention of 70% of revenue is reasonable to cover the overhead of the practice. The analysis of the appropriateness of the arrangement must include consideration of the fact that, with respect to surgical services, most of the related overhead is being borne by the ASC, not the practice.

In addition to the issues discussed above, the arrangement could raise concerns under state fee-split prohibitions. Although some state medical boards are not inclined to challenge the propriety of percentage-based compensation arrangements when such arrangements occur within physician group practices, other boards find these kinds of terms to be inappropriate, even within the context of a group practice.

Aside from restructuring the arrangement to comply with the reassignment rules and to avoid the anti-kickback and fee split risks, there is one alternative consideration. Both the reassignment rules and the anti-kickback statutes have exceptions for *bona fide* employees. Similarly, state fee-split prohibitions generally do not apply to employees of a physician practice. Therefore, if the parties were willing, the retina specialist could become an employee of the practice under the same financial terms as outlined above.

40

MULTIPLE OFFICE GROUP PRACTICE

Nine ophthalmologists, comprising three separate practices, decide to combine to form a larger group practice. The combined group will continue to practice at all three locations, with three ophthalmologists working principally at each of the separate office locations. The members of the group agree that each member shall be compensated on the basis of his or her own individual collections, minus an allocation of the expenses for the office wher he or she works. In addition, each ophthalmologist will receive the net profits from the A-scans, B-scans, and postcataract lenses and spectacles that he or she orders.

IS THERE ANY LIMITATION ON THE WAY PHYSICIANS MAY STRUCTURE A COMPENSATION RELATIONSHIP WITHIN THEIR PRACTICE?

The major issue for this arrangement is compliance with the federal Physician Anti-Self-Referral Law, also known as the Stark Law. The Stark Law prohibits physicians from referring Medicare or Medicaid patients for certain "designated health services" to an entity with which they have a financial relationship. Among the designated health services are radiology services, including magnetic resonance imaging, computerized axial tomography scans, and ultrasound services. Radiology services include A-scans and B-scans.

Under the Stark Law, a physician has made a referral simply by ordering a service. Thus, when physicians order A-scans and B-scans, the Stark Law is triggered, and the physicians would be prohibited from making such a referral even within the practice, unless an exception to the Stark Law applies. The relevant exception is one for the provision of "in-office ancillary service," which requires that the services be provided by, or under, the supervision of a physician who is a member of the group practice. Although this requirement appears simple and straightforward, it is not; the Stark Law has a detailed and restrictive definition of what qualifies as a *group practice*.

First, in order to qualify as a *group practice* under the Stark Law, a practice must function as an integrated, "unified" business and not merely as separate practices bound together in name or referrals alone. In the proposed regulation published by the Center for Medicare and Medicaid Services (CMS), this practice's site-by-site allocation of expenses would have caused concern, as CMS initially had taken the position that an entity could not be a unified business if it shared expenses based on "cost centers." In response to criticism that the proposed regulation would have excluded many bona fide group practices and intruded too far into the financial operations of physician practices, CMS substantially revised the group practice definition in the final rule, and separate cost-centers are permitted. However, a group practice still must be organized and operated on a bona fide basis, as a single integrated business enterprise with legal and organizational integration, among other requirements. There are additional requirements that must be met for the group to qualify as a group practice, including:

- ✧ Each physician who is a member of the group must substantially offer the "full range of patient care services" that the physician routinely furnishes, including medical care, consultation, diagnosis, and treatment, through the joint use of shared office space, facilities, equipment, and personnel.

- ✧ At least 75% of the total patient care services of the group practice members must be furnished through the group and billed under a billing number assigned to the group, and the amounts received must be treated as receipts of the group.

- ✧ The overhead expenses and income from the practice must be distributed according to methods that are determined before the receipt of payment for the services giving rise to the overhead expense or producing the income.

- ✧ Members of the group must personally conduct no less than 75% of the physician-patient encounters of the group practice.

The group practice definition also imposes certain limitations on how physician compensation may be determined. Specifically, the physician members of a group are prohibited from directly receiving compensation based on the volume or value of their own referrals, unless they perform the services themselves or the services are *incident to* the individual physician's services. Applying this limitation to the fact pattern described above, the law permits the group practice to compensate the physicians based on their collections, reduced by an allocation of expenses to reflect the overhead of their office. Unless the physicians personally perform the A-scans or B-scans, however, because these services are designated health services, the proposed compensation methodology is not acceptable under Stark. Instead, profits derived from designated health services must be distributed equally in a manner that does not reflect the volume or value of referrals for such services, such as sharing those profits.

Finally, payment of a bonus based on the volume of postcataract spectacles ordered is permissible under the Stark Law. Despite the technical categorization of postcataract surgery spectacles as a "prosthetic device," and therefore a designated health service under Stark, CMS exempted post-cataract spectacles from the list of designated health services under the final regulations.

41

CREDIT BALANCES

An ophthalmologist becomes concerned that his practice administrator is not performing adequately and decides to hire a new administrator. The new administrator is asked to evaluate the practice during the first 2 weeks of her employment in a thorough fashion and report any issues to the ophthalmologist. Two days later, the new administrator comes into the ophthalmologist's office and reports that the practice has accumulated credit balances in the amount of $27,534.32. Some of the credit balances date back as long as 5 years. Apparently, the prior administrator had not instituted any system to return or otherwise dispose of credit balances. The ophthalmologist asks the administrator what should be done.

HOW SHOULD A PRACTICE TREAT CREDIT BALANCES?

The answer, painful as it may be, is that the practice needs to take steps to return the overpayments. To the extent that the credit balances reflect Medicare and Medicaid services, the law makes it a criminal violation for any person to fail to disclose or refund a known overpayment of Medicare or Medicaid monies. Further, the federal government has pursued cases involving credit balances that were taken into income by a provider. In these cases, the goverment alleged that the providers had committed a criminal conversion (or theft) of government property.

Overpayments related to private payor and self-pay services can raise similar issues. The federal government has taken action against some providers for failing to return copayment and deductible amounts collected in error from Medicare beneficiaries and retained by the providers. Under state law, insurance fraud provisions may require the disclosure or refund of the overpayments. Private payor agreements may require the prompt refund of overpayments, such that a state law fraud claim may be brought by a payor whose money is not returned.

Unfortunately, various complications can be encountered when trying to return overpayments. Situations where Medicare carriers, as well as private payors, have returned refunded overpayments are common. In order to prevent being later accused of fraud for failure to make the refund, physicians should attempt to make the refund in writing *at least twice* by certified mail. Copies of the letters should be retained in the files for future reference.

Some private payors may have provisions in their provider agreements that make all payment decisions final after a certain period of time, meaning generally that a provider may retain an amount that was paid in error. Physicians are cautioned that failure to refund overpayments *identified* within the prescribed period, but held until after expiration of the time limit for refund, may result in an allegation of fraud. If the overpayment is identified only after the end of the identified period, we still suggest considering sending a letter that notifies the payor of the overpayment but states that the funds will be retained, as permitted by the contract, unless the payor provides documentation to support the repayment.

There also may be problems when a practice tries to make a refund to a patient. A patient may have moved with no forwarding address or may have died. A practice generally is not entitled to retain a patient overpayment, even under these circumstances. Many states have something called an Escheat Law, where, if a person or entity cannot find the rightful owner of funds or other property after a specified period of time, they are obligated to turn the property over to the state. The state then attempts to find the owner of the property. After a fixed period of time, if the owner has not been located—you guessed it—the state takes the property.

In summary, a practice should take immediate steps to return known overpayments to the appropriate party and should have procedures in place to assure their prompt identification and refund.

42

REFUND OF OVERPAYMENT

During a routine self-audit, the compliance officer for an ophthalmology practice discovered that the practice has been submitting claims for a particular service using the incorrect CPT code. An internal investigation by the billing supervisor revealed that the error was due to a misunderstanding among the staff, and as a result, the practice was paid more than it should have been for the service at issue.

WHAT IS THE PRACTICE'S RESPONSIBILITY TO THE MEDICARE PROGRAM WHEN IT DISCOVERS IT HAS BEEN OVERPAID?

An overpayment is any amount a physician or beneficiary receives in excess of the amount payable under the Medicare program. The Medicare Carriers Manual specifically provides that physicians are liable for overpayments, even if the overpayment is the result of an error by a Medicare carrier. Except in certain instances, where an overpayment is more than 3 years old and was not due to any fault of the physician, overpayments are considered a debt to the United States and must be repaid.

In the scenario above, the practice's compliance officer should undertake or oversee an organized review of all the claims submitted to Medicare that involve the service in question to verify whether the claims were coded appropriately and, if not, the extent of an overpayment. Once a physician knows that he or she has been overpaid, the carrier should be notified immediately in writing. The letter should set out the basis for the overpayment, the fact that it was identified through an internal compliance review, and, if possible, identify the patients affected and dates of service. The letter should include a check for the entire amount of the overpayment or, if the practice is not in a position to repay the entire amount, a partial payment should be enclosed with a proposal for making payment over time. Be prepared, however, for the carrier to respond with a demand for financial information relating to the practice's ability to pay, and the imposition of an interest amount on the outstanding balance in excess of 13%. Practices would be wise to borrow funds from the bank to avoid high interest rates and burdensome Medicare repayment schedules. Finally, the practice also must develop a mechanism to refund private payors and patients in connection with improper co-payments.

CHARGING FOR
NON-MEDICARE PATIENTS
AT LESS THAN THE MEDICARE RATE

A practice decides that it does not want to make contractual adjustments after receiving payments from its various payors. A contractual adjustment is the write-off that a practice takes after it is paid by a payor to reflect the difference between the provider's charges and the allowable that has been paid. Accordingly, the practice abandons its single fee schedule and develops one that, for each payor, makes the applicable charge what that payor will accept as the maximum allowable. Because the practice is located in an area where there is a heavy penetration of managed care providers, charges for more than 50% of the practice's patients under this system will be significantly lower than the Medicare allowable for the service.

MAY THE PRACTICE BILL FOR
NON-MEDICARE PATIENTS AT A SIGNIFICANT
DISCOUNT FROM THE MEDICARE CHARGE?

The Medicare statute contains a prohibition against a physician or provider from charging the Medicare program an amount substantially in excess of the practice's usual charge. The penalty for violating this provision is exclusion from the Medicare and Medicaid programs. Unfortunately, there has been no formal guidance from the Office of the Inspector General or the Center for Medicare and Medicaid Services (CMS) concerning the standards to apply in determining how much is "substantially in excess" and what constitutes a practice's "usual charge." As a result, practices have had to rely on common sense and the limited informal guidance that has developed over the years.

The more significant issue is what constitutes a practice's usual charge. It has been generally recognized that the usual charge is the amount charged to the practice's typical patient. Thus, if a practice charges a rate to the majority of its patients, it likely would be considered a practice's usual charge. In this case, however, the majority of the patients are covered by managed care programs. According to informal opinions from the former Health Care Financing Administration (now CMS), the managed care population is not considered when a practice's usual charge is determined. Instead, it appears that the Medicare program would limit its consideration to patients who are not covered by managed care programs.

Therefore, in this example, even though the practice's charge to a majority of its patients may be substantially below the Medicare charge, it appears that the statutory prohibition would not be triggered as long as the charge to the majority of nonmanaged care patients is consistent with the Medicare charge.

With respect to the question of what constitutes "substantially in excess," there is absolutely no guidance. Here, common sense must dictate a practice's pricing decisions. If Medicare were charged a premium above all other payors, the government undoubtedly would view such conduct unfavorably and would argue that even a modest premium could constitute "substantially in excess." On the other hand, if the practice's charges varied widely and there were no Medicare premium pricing, such a position by the government would be less likely.

There is one final consideration with respect to this issue. The government has never pursued an exclusion action against a physician for such conduct. Although that fact should provide some comfort, it is important to be sensitive to the statutory prohibition. No physician wants to be the test case.

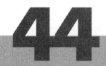

ADVANCED BENEFICIARY NOTICES

Ophthalmology specialists (OS) offers a particular diagnostic test to certain patients, and while the physicians in the group believe the test is medically necessary for this patient population, the Medicare carrier generally denies payment for the service. There is no national coverage determination regarding the test, nor a local medical review policy. In order to protect itself, OS requires every Medicare beneficiary who wants to undergo the study to sign an advanced beneficiary notice (ABN). The ABN informs the patient that Medicare may deny payment for the test on the grounds that it was not medically necessary, and that if Medicare should refuse coverage, the patient is responsible for paying the fee for the test.

IS THIS A PROPER USE OF AN ABN?

Medicare protects beneficiaries from liability for claims that are denied because the medical care is deemed to be not medically necessary, if the beneficiary did not know, and had no reason to know, that the care was not medically necessary.

In deciding whether a beneficiary knew or could reasonably be expected to have known that an item or service he or she received was not reasonable and necessary, Medicare carriers will accept a beneficiary's allegation that he or she did not know in the absence of evidence that rebuts the beneficiary's position. ABNs are forms that allow a physician to document that a beneficiary was informed in writing that Medicare likely would not pay for an item or service before the service was furnished and that the beneficiary agreed to pay the physician for the service if Medicare will not.

To be considered adequate notice, an ABN must (1) be provided to the patient *before the excluded item or service is performed*; (2) describe the particular service(s) involved; and (3) contain the physician's reasons for believing Medicare will deny payment.

Because an ABN must describe the item or service and the reason for the expected denial with some specificity, the requirement for advance notice is not satisfied by a signed statement that states only that there is a possibility that Medicare may not pay for the service.

In the situation described above, OS reasonably could be expected to know that the carrier would deny payment for the diagnostic test at issue. Therefore, in order to shift liability for the cost of the test from OS to the patient benefiting from the test, OS must provide an ABN to each patient for whom the test is recommended before furnishing the test. To be certain it provides sufficient notice, OS should use the ABN developed and approved by the Center for Medicare and Medicaid Services (CMS) for use with Part B services. The ABN (Form CMS-R-131-G) may be downloaded from the CMS website at: www.hcfa.gov/medlearn/refabn.htm.

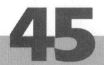

A group of investors own an ambulatory surgical center (ASC) The ASC is Medicare certified and provides Medicare ASC covered list services, including cataract surgery. In addition, the ASC provides laser assisted in situ keratomileusis (LASIK) and other surgical services that are not on the Medicare ASC approved list. The ASC is not as busy as the investors had planned, and in order to generate additional revenue, the investors decide to rent out part of the ASC-certified space for several ophthalmologists to perform consults. The leases are at arm's length, reflect fair market value, and fit within the space lease safe harbor.

DOES LEASING SPACE IN THE ASC TO PHYSICIANS WHO PERFORM NONSURGICAL SERVICES AFFECT THE ASC'S CERTIFICATION?

In order to participate in the Medicare program, a facility must meet the Medicare definition of an ASC. The Medicare regulations define an ASC as "any distinct entity that operates *exclusively* for the purpose of providing surgical services to patients not requiring hospitalization" and that meets other regulatory requirements. If an ASC is not a distinct entity nor operating exclusively for the purpose of providing surgical services, as the Center for Medicare and Medicaid Services (CMS) interprets these terms, the ASC will no longer meet the Medicare definition. If a facility no longer meets the Medicare definition of an ASC, the ASC cannot be Medicare certified. If a facility is not Medicare certified, then Medicare will not reimburse the ASC for surgery performed on Medicare patients.

By applying the Medicare definition to the above scenario, the ASC would not meet the Medicare definition of an ASC. By permitting ophthalmologists to lease part of the certified space for consultations, the ASC no longer operates *exclusively* for the purpose of providing surgical services. In order to maintain the rental arrangement and meet the definition, the ASC must "carve out" the areas of rented space completely from the certified facility, as long as the "carve out" does not otherwise adversely impact the certification. To avoid uncertainty, inquiry should be made with the appropriate state survey agency.

Until recently, the facts set forth above would have triggered a second issue based on the provision of non-ASC list covered procedures (eg, LASIK) in addition to ASC list covered procedures. Specifically, some officials in CMS had expressed the view that the provision of non-ASC list covered procedures by an ASC also would jeopardize the ASC's Medicare-certification. In fact, however, CMS recently confirmed that Medicare certified ASCs may provide surgical services that are not Medicare ASC list procedures, as Medicare requires that an ASC be operated for the purpose of providing *surgical* services; it is not limited to *covered* surgical services or services on the ASC list.

SUPERVISION OF DIAGNOSTIC TESTS

Dr. Jones is a solo practitioner who specializes in cataract surgery. In order to increase the efficiency of her practice and give patients more flexibility in scheduling appointments for diagnostic tests—including B-scans (CPT codes 76512 and 76513), Dr. Jones schedules her ophthalmic technician, Ms. Young, to be in the office 5 days a week to perform such tests. Because Dr. Jones has tremendous confidence in Ms. Young's clinical and technical skills, Dr. Jones permits Ms. Young to perform these tests while Dr. Jones is at the hospital performing surgery. One day while scrubbing for her next case, Dr. Jones began talking with Dr. Sheehan, another ophthalmologist who performs surgery at the same hospital, about the difficulties of running a solo practice and how she relies on Ms. Young a great deal. Dr. Sheehan informs Dr. Jones that based on information he received at a recent lecture on fraud and abuse, he thinks she might be violating Medicare rules by allowing Ms. Young to perform the scans when Dr. Jones is not in the office.

IS DR. SHEEHAN CORRECT?

Yes. When Dr. Jones submits claims for the scans she did not supervise directly, she is violating the Medicare coverage and payment rules, as well as the federal Physician Anti-Self-Referral Act, more commonly referred to as the Stark Law.

Diagnostic tests covered under the Medicare Physician Fee Schedule must be performed, with certain exceptions, under the supervision of a physician in order to be covered by Medicare. The Medicare coverage and payment rules require that B-scans described by CPT codes 76512 and 76513 be performed under the direct supervision of a physician. This means that in order for B-scans to be payable, the physician must be in the office suite and immediately available to furnish assistance and direction throughout the performance of the procedure.

In addition to the supervision requirement relating to reimbursement, the Stark Law has supervision requirements as well. The Stark Law prohibits a physician from ordering a service that is provided by an entity with which the physician or an immediate family member has a financial relationship if the service falls within one of the categories of designated health services (DHS) covered by the Stark Law and is reimbursed by Medicare or Medicaid, and if the financial relationship does not qualify for an exception. The DHS covered by the law includes B-scans among other diagnostic imaging services such as CT scans, MRI, and ultrasound. Penalties for violating the Stark Law include forfeiture of any reimbursement for services rendered based on an unlawful referral, civil fines of up to $15,000 per violation, and exclusion from the Medicare and Medicaid programs.

Because of the broad scope of the Stark Law, Congress exempted certain types of referrals from the self-referral prohibition and authorized the Secretary of the US Department of Health and Human Services to except, by regulation, other arrangements the department believes pose little fraud and abuse risk. A referral that otherwise implicates the Stark Law must fall within a statutory or regulatory exception or it is, per se, illegal.

Referrals for a DHS, even within a solo practice, trigger the Stark Law. Congress, however, recognized that it may be cost-efficient and convenient for Medicare beneficiaries to obtain certain DHS at their doctor's office, and, therefore, crafted the "in-office ancillary services" exception that permits referrals for DHS performed within a physician's own practice. Under this exception, referrals such as the one Dr. Jones makes for the B-scan are permitted so long as a number of criteria are met. One such criterion is that the DHS must be furnished personally by the referring physician, a member of the same group practice as the referring physician, or by an *individual who is supervised by the referring physician* or by another physician in the group practice.

In determining what level of physician supervision, either general, direct, or personal, is required an individual furnishing a DHS to a Medicare beneficiary must be under for the purpose of meeting the terms of the in-office ancillary services exception, the Stark Law defers to the Medicare coverage and payment rules. Because

Medicare has determined that B-scans represented by CPT codes 76512 and 76513 must be performed under a physician's direct supervision in order to be covered, this same standard applies when deciding whether a referral qualifies for the in-office ancillary exception.

PATIENT TRANSPORTATION

An ophthalmology practice is located in a small city in a generally rural state. Approximately half of the practice's patients come from the small city and its immediate surrounding areas; the remaining half come from up to 75 miles beyond the city environs. In order to accommodate all of its patients, the practice provides van transportation service. While originally designed for patients from the rural areas, the practice provides the service to any patient who requests it. There is no active promotion of the transportation services by any of the practice's employees. Only after patients have scheduled their appointment with the practice are they asked whether they have transportation services available or whether they are needed. However, in its yellow pages advertisement, there is a picture of the practice's van with the practice's name on the side, and the statement "Transportation Services Available."

IS IT APPROPRIATE TO PROVIDE TRANSPORTATION SERVICES FOR PATIENTS?

The issue of the propriety of providing transportation services to patients has been debated for many years. Several years ago, at a congressional hearing, a question was raised to the Inspector General of the Department of Health and Human Services whether such conduct could be considered a violation of the Anti-Kickback Statute. When the Inspector General responded that he did not feel such conduct clearly fit into the prohibitions of the statute, the issue appeared to die. However, in 1996, Congress passed the Health Insurance Portability and Accountability Act (HIPAA), which included, among several antifraud and abuse provisions, a section of the law that is known as the Patient Inducement Prohibition. Under HIPAA, it is a civil violation for any provider of services to offer a patient anything of value that the provider knows or should have known would induce the patient to select that provider of services over another. Recognizing that such a broad prohibition could discourage beneficial services that should be encouraged, the Conference Committee Report that accompanied HIPAA included language clarifying that the statute was not meant to discourage items of nominal value, such as participation in free health fairs, medical literature, and complimentary local transportation services. The key question to be addressed, therefore, is whether the facts set forth above could be viewed to violate the Patient Inducement Prohibition. The analysis focuses on two issues: (1) whether or not the transportation services described could be deemed as "beneficial services," as presented in the report language; or (2) whether the transportation services described above could be deemed not to be an inducement, and therefore, does not trigger the statute.

With respect to the beneficial services question, there is, unfortunately, no definition of "local transportation services," nor is there a definition of "nominal" value. While 75 miles would not generally be considered local, if the practice routinely attracts patients from that radius, and 75 miles constitutes the practice's local catchment area, it may qualify as local. Similarly, while roundtrip cab fare for a 75-mile trip would likely be beyond what is considered a nominal amount, a roundtrip bus ticket for the same distance may, in fact, be considered nominal.

The more important analysis, however, is the question of whether the transportation services described are, in fact, an inducement that could trigger the statutory prohibition. To fall under the statute, an inducement likely would require that there be an offer of something of value in order to convince a patient to select a particular practice. In this case, however, the offer of transportation services is made only *after* the patient has already scheduled an appointment with the practice. In such a case, it is difficult to argue that the transportation services constituted an inducement. Further, the fact that there is no active promotion of the transportation services by any employee of the practice also supports the position that there is no inducement. The only potential problem is the yellow pages advertisement. A patient looking for an ophthalmologist in the yellow pages may well be influenced to select a particular practice by the availability of transportation services. Therefore, to avoid an allegation that the transportation services constituted a prohibited inducement, the practice should eliminate any reference in their yellow pages advertisement.

The general issue of providing transportation services to patients has been addressed in an Advisory Opinion published by the Office of the Inspector General (OIG) in November 2000—OIG *Advisory Opinion No. 00-7*. In that case, a hospital offered transportation services for a group of patients receiving extended courses of treatment at the hospital. In its opinion approving the services, the OIG identified a series of factors that it considered relevant, including:

 ✧ The nature of the free transportation (ie, airline, limousine, or van)
 ✧ The geographic area where the services are offered (ie, within or outside of the provider's historic service area)
 ✧ Whether the free transportation services are marketed
 ✧ Whether the cost of the services will be claimed directly or indirectly on a federal health care program cost report
 ✧ The limited availability of publicly available and economical transportation services

At the same time, the OIG indicated that providing transportation services to all patients is a factor that would not be viewed favorably.

In this case, the reasonableness of the service is supported by the modest mode of transportation offered (van service), the limitation to the practice's catchment area, the provision of service to a rural area, the fact that employees do not promote the service, and the fact that the cost of the services are not claimed on a cost report. The practice should, however, eliminate the yellow pages advertisement to reduce the risk of an allegation of inducement. While it may not be necessary, restricting the availability of services to a group of infirm patients, such as those who continue to have visual disability, would reduce the risk still further.

PROFESSIONAL COURTESY

Quality Ophthalmology, P.C. (QO) extends professional courtesy discounts to ophthalmologists and optometrists who are in active practice within a 50-mile radius of QO, as well the families of these providers. QO's professional courtesy policy consists of waiving any coinsurance obligation an ophthalmologist, optometrist, or family member may be required to pay by Medicare or any private third-party payor (ie, "insurance-only" billing). Some, but not all, of the recipients of QO's professional courtesy policy refer patients to QO.

DOES QO's PROFESSIONAL COURTESY POLICY PLACE THE PRACTICE AT RISK?

Professional courtesy may raise fraud and abuse concerns, particularly when recipients of professional courtesy are selected in a manner that directly or indirectly takes into account their ability to affect referrals, or otherwise generate business for the physician offering the free or discounted service. Where Medicare services are involved, both the federal Anti-Kickback Statute and the Patient Inducement Prohibition may be implicated. If the professional courtesy extends to services paid for by commercial insurers, state anti-kickback and insurance fraud laws may be triggered.

In its Model Compliance Program for Individual and Small Group Physician Practices, the Office of the Inspector General (OIG) set forth guidance regarding professional courtesy. According to the OIG, a physician's risk of violating the federal Anti-Kickback Statute is reduced significantly when a physician has a regular and consistent policy of extending professional courtesy to both referral and nonreferral sources and in a manner that does not take ability to refer into account. In fact, the OIG stated that physicians who regularly waive the entire service fee to a group of persons might not implicate the fraud and abuse laws. These waivers are acceptable as long as membership in the group receiving the courtesy is not based on a person's ability to refer patients to the physician either directly or indirectly. The legality of any professional courtesy arrangement, however, will depend on the specific facts presented, and in respect to allegations that a physician violated the Anti-Kickback Statute, on the specific intent of the parties involved.

Aside from the issue of whether the Anti-Kickback Statute is triggered, the OIG made it clear in the model program, and again in a 2001 Advisory Opinion that, except in circumstances of documented patient financial hardship, any waiver of a Medicare copayment is viewed as an improper patient inducement because it is likely to influence a beneficiary's decision as to where to receive services.

QO's professional courtesy policy raises some concern and should be modified. The government could allege that by extending professional courtesy only to those ophthalmologists and optometrists in active practice located within a 50-mile radius of QO, the policy is designed to limit professional courtesy to those who are likely to be referral sources. The policy instead should eliminate any geographic restrictions and should apply equally to all physicians and optometrists, regardless of whether they are in active practice or retired. Furthermore, QO's policy of insurance-only billing runs the risk that it may run afoul of the Patient Inducement Prohibition. QO could eliminate this risk by implementing a policy to waive the entire fee rather than the just any requisite copayments. Insurance-only billing should be limited to financial, not courtesy, considerations.

49

SALE OF FREE SAMPLES

Eye Associates (EA) is a busy ophthalmology practice specializing in the treatment of glaucoma and cataract surgery. Every year EA receives free drug samples from a sales representative for Pharmaceutical U.S.A., Inc. In the last several years, the value of the free samples totaled nearly $6000 annually. Many of these free samples are often given to needy patients. However, at the urging of the sales representative (who provides more samples than EA requires), the practice often sells the samples to patients to help make up for the continuing decline in Medicare payments.

IS EA AT ANY LEGAL RISK FOR SELLING THE FREE SAMPLES TO PATIENTS?

Yes. EA may be liable under the federal Food, Drug, and Cosmetic Act (FDCA) as well as both the federal and state anti-kickback laws.

The FDCA is enforced by the U.S. Food and Drug Administration. The FDCA prohibits the sale, purchase, or trade, or the offer to sell, purchase, or trade drug samples. For purposes of this provision, a drug sample is defined as a unit of drug that is not intended to be sold and is intended to promote the sale of the drug. Drug samples generally are labeled as samples that are not for resale. Violations of the FDCA are punishable by fines and/or imprisonment.

The sale of the free samples to patients also raises significant risk that EA could be liable for receiving an illegal kickback. For example, the federal Anti-Kickback Statute makes it a crime to knowingly offer, pay, solicit, or receive anything of value (direct or indirect, overt or covert, in cash or in kind) that is intended to induce the referral of a patient for an item or service that is reimbursed by a federal health care program, including Medicare, Medicaid, TRI-

CARE, and the programs covering veterans' benefits. The law ascribes liability to both sides of an impermissible kickback transaction and has been interpreted broadly by several courts to apply to situations where only one purpose of a payment is to induce referrals, notwithstanding the fact that there may be other legitimate purposes for which the payment is made.

Traditional application of the Anti-Kickback Statute involves cases in which physicians are paid some type of remuneration to refer patients to another health care provider or entity. However, the law also applies to a physician or other health care provider who is paid remuneration to prescribe or otherwise recommend a drug that is covered by a federal health care program. Assuming EA treats Medicare beneficiaries or Medicaid recipients and prescribes medications or orders items that are manufactured by Pharmaceutical U.S.A, Inc. and are paid for by federal health care program, then the additional "samples" could be viewed as a kickback for prescribing Pharmaceutical U.S.A. products. If such an intent could be shown, the Anti-Kickback Statute would be implicated.

Even if EA were not ordering medications or items that were covered and paid for by a federal health care program, EA is not necessarily free from legal risk. Many states have passed anti-kickback laws that mirror the prohibition found in the federal statute but which apply to items and services paid for by any payor including the patient (these statutes are referred to as *all-payor anti-kickback laws*). Like the federal statute, these laws may carry civil and/or criminal penalties such as fines and imprisonment or administrative sanctions against a physician's medical license.

SOPHISTICATED CLAIMS
PROCESSING SOFTWARE

FACTS

An ophthalmology practice has continuing problems with its claims submissions and experiences significant denials by the Medicare carrier and private insurers. Its physicians are rushed and do not fill out their superbills completely, the billing department has been suffering from constant turnover, its billing staff is inexperienced and untrained, and the local Medicare carrier is constantly changing its policies and tightening its systems. In a professional society meeting, the physicians are attracted to an exhibitor promoting claims processing software. Marketed as "the closest thing to being idiot-proof," the software is designed to minimize all of the kinds of problems the physicians have been facing. One function, which is particularly intriguing, includes a default system that will automatically reject any diagnosis code that does not support the procedure billed and replace it with the most common code used by ophthalmologists for that particular procedure. The ophthalmologists think this may be the answer they have been seeking.

CAN THIS SOFTWARE PACKAGE SOLVE
THE OPHTHALMOLOGIST'S PROBLEMS?

While this software billing package may solve the ophthalmologist's problem of excessive denials, it could create a far bigger one: the risk of filing false claims. When a claim is submitted for reimbursement, it is not only a statement of what was done (through the CPT code) but is also a statement of why a service was performed (through the ICD-9 code). Only the physician is in a position to state why a particular procedure or service was performed. If the physician enters an ICD-9 code and the software program changes it to a code that will assure that the claim will be paid, it is likely that the government will take the position that the physician has caused a false claim to be submitted and could subject the practice to treble (ie, tripled) damages and penalties.

The concept of manipulating the ICD-9 code to assure that a claim is paid has been described as *code steering* or *code stuffing*. In the mid-1990s, there were a series of federal investigations of clinical laboratories that were accused of advising physicians which codes should be used in order to assure reimbursement of clinical laboratory services (code steering). Physicians were also reportedly advised in cases where the wrong code or no code was used, in which case the laboratory would file the claim using a code designed to assure payment (code stuffing). Each of these investigations resulted in significant settlement payments by the laboratories. Physicians who employ software that manipulates the ICD-9 code to assure payment could be subject to similar risk of False Claims Act liability.

Facts

A pharmaceutical company (the Company) has a breakthrough product that has just been approved for Medicare reimbursement. Dr. Smith was one of the drug's clinical investigators and believes that the drug is a significant advancement that will greatly benefit ophthalmic patients worldwide. Dr. Smith is well known and very well respected in his subspecialty. He is approached by the Company to give a presentation sharing his experience as an investigator relating to the product at a worldwide ophthalmological conference in Paris, France. The Company offers to pay for Dr. Smith's expenses, including first-class airfare from his home in Chicago, meals, a week's stay at a hotel in Paris, plus an honorarium of $10,000. The Company is careful not to interfere in any way with the content or conclusion of Dr. Smith's presentation.

May Dr. Smith Accept the Company's Offer?

Relations between physicians and pharmaceutical companies are targets for examination and enforcement by government authorities. Important recent enforcement developments include the TAP Pharmaceuticals investigation and settlement, as well as the HHS Office of Inspector General's (OIG) FY 2002 Work Plan.

In particular, the OIG work plan indicates that the OIG plans to increase its focus on the relationships between physicians and pharmaceutical companies. The OIG is concerned about such companies providing anything of value to physicians and other health care providers as an inducement to order company products. In the view of the OIG, such conduct creates both inherent conflicts of interest as well as potential violations of the federal Anti-Kickback Statute. The federal Anti-Kickback Statute prohibits the knowing offer or receipt of anything of value in exchange for referring, recommending, or arranging for a product or service paid for by a federal health care program.

Not all physician relationships with pharmaceutical companies are prohibited or inappropriate, however. To avoid unreasonable risks, several basic principles should be followed. For example, with respect to receipt of anything of value in return for presenting at conferences, individuals who are meeting faculty, company consultants, or researchers may receive reasonable compensation for services rendered. These services should be provided pursuant to an appropriate written contract. It also is appropriate for compensation from pharmaceutical companies for such personal services to include reasonable travel costs and either an honorarium or payment for the faculty member's time. Payment should reflect fair market value for the physician's time, recognizing that the time involved includes preparation of the presentation and travel away from one's practice, in addition to the actual presentation itself. If a physician believes that the benefits received exceed the value of the contribution made, the physician should consider a reevaluation of the relationship. Further, physicians should at all times retain responsibility and control over the content of their lecture.

Applying these principles, the above example raises issues for Dr. Smith as well as the Company. Even assuming that both the conference and Dr. Smith's presentation are of bona fide value, and the content of his presentation is solely under his control, payment must reflect reasonable fair market value for services provided. The Paris location, the first-class airline ticket, and the four-star hotel all serve to heighten the scrutiny of enforcement officials. These alone, however, are unlikely to trigger any accusation that the Anti-Kickback Statute has been violated. Two aspects of the arrangement, however, may raise questions.

First, covering 1 week at a four-star hotel when Dr. Smith appears to be making a single 45-minute presentation may raise questions, particularly if Dr. Smith's spouse accompanies him to Paris, and the couple spent the remainder of the week sightseeing. On the other hand, if Dr. Smith remains at the conference and continues to confer with other physicians about the new drug, the week-long stay would be appropriate.

Similarly, the $10,000 honorarium appears high for a 45-minute presentation but, again, this presumably covers preparation time, as well as lost time away from Dr. Smith's practice. The key to defending the propriety of the honorarium is to be able to document the time spent by Dr. Smith on behalf of the Company and to demonstrate that the honorarium reflects fair market value for that time.

INDEX

Advance beneficiary notice (ABN), 34
    proper use of, 103–104
Advertisement
    acceptable copy in, 63–64
    of patient transportation services, 111, 112
All-payor anti-kickback laws, 118
Ambulatory surgery center list covered proce-
    dures, 105
Ambulatory surgery centers
    investing in, 83–85
    Medicare certification of, 105–106
Anti-Kickback Statute, 74, 80
    changing referral pattern and, 82
    on compensating physician independent
        contractors, 91–92
    exceptions to, 88–89
    leasing agreements and, 77–78
    physician-pharmaceutical company rela-
        tionships under, 121–122
    professional courtesy and, 115–116
    on remuneration for referrals, 83–85
    safe harbor to, 83–84, 89
    on sale of free samples, 117–118
    on self-referrals, 88–90
    transportation services under, 111–112
Argon laser trabeculoplasty, examination on day
    of, 13

B-scans, supervision of, 107–109
Beneficial services, prohibition of, 111–113
Billing. *See also* Fees
    for argon focal laser and initial panretinal
        photocoagulation, 27–28
    for consultations within group practice, 7–8
    for examination on day of surgical procedure, 13
    for extended ophthalmoscopy, 37–38
    improper use of physician PIN numbers for, 5–6
    for LASIK, 79–80
    by multiple office group practices, 94–95
    for new patient visit, 3
    for new technology, 31–32
    of non-Medicare patients, 101–102
    for optical dispensary, 33–34
    for physician face-to-face time, 29–30
    for physician subcontractor services, 91–92
    responsibility for accuracy of, 67–68

software package for, 119–120
    using incorrect CPT code, 99–100
    of visual field testing for glaucoma patient,
        9–10
Blepharoplasty surgery, documenting, 23–24
Brightness acuity test (BAT), 45, 46
Bundling, 35–36

Carriers, coding advice from, 55–56
Carve outs, nonsurgical service, 106
Cataract surgery
    patient qualification for, 45–46
    second, 43–44
Center for Medicare and Medicaid Services (CMS)
    advanced beneficiary notice of, 104
    E/M service documentation guidelines for, 47–49
    multiple office group practices under, 94–95
    national Correct Coding Initiative of, 35–36
    optical services policies of, 34
    Stark II regulations of, 87–88
Charts
    documentation requirement guidelines in,
        51–52
    notation requirements in, 51–52
Child examination, chart notation require-
    ments in, 51–52
Civil False Claims Act, 68
Claims
    physician's responsibility for accuracy of, 67–68
    processing software for, 119–120
    review of for incorrect CPT code, 99–100
Code 67228, 27–28
Code 92135, 11–12
Code 92225/92226, misunderstanding of, 37
Code steering/stuffing, 120
Coding
    documentation of carrier advice on, 55–56
    Medicare utilization data identifying issues
        in, 59–60
Collagen plugs, overutilization of, 61–62
Comanagement arrangements
    commercial insurance covering services in, 75–76
    ophthalmologist-optometrist contracts in, 73–74
    for refractive surgery, 81–82
Compensation relationships, structuring of,
    93–95

Investigational procedures, Medicare coverage of, 31-32
Investments, safe harbor protection for, 84–85

Joint Venture Arrangements under the Anti-Kickback Statute, Fraud Alert on, 89–90
Joint ventures, legal risks of, 87–90

Kickbacks, 80
ambulatory surgery center investment and, 83–85
from joint ventures, 88–90
legal issues of, 74
for physician independent contractors, 91–92
for refractive surgery referrals, 82
sale of free samples as, 117–118

Laser surgery, off-label use of, 69
LASIK, billing issues related to, 79–80
Lease agreements
for nonsurgical services, 105–106
between ophthalmologist and optometrist, 77–78
safe harbor for, 78
Legal issues, 73–123
Lifestyle problems, documenting, 23–24
Local Medical Review Policies (LMRP), 9–10
on extended ophthalmoscopy, 37

Managed care programs, fee charged to, 102
Marketing, acceptable ad copy in, 63–64
Medical necessity
justification for, 45–46
overutilization of procedures and, 61–62
of postoperative YAG capsulotomies, 57–58
Medical records
guidelines for requirements in, 51–52
responsibility for accuracy of, 67–68
support for E/M service claims in, 47–49
Medicare
advance beneficiary notice of payment denial by, 103–104
annual glaucoma screening under, 15–16
certification of ambulatory surgery centers, 105–106
charging higher rates, 101–102
consultation defined by, 39–40
investigational procedures under, 31–32
Local Medical Review Policies of, 9–10
"new patient" defined by, 3
optical dispensary coverage under, 33–34
Physician Fee Schedule on supervision of diagnostic testing, 107–109
reasonable and medical necessity requirement of, 43–44, 45–46
reassignment rules of, 73–74
reassignment rules of for physician independent contractors, 91–92
repayment schedules and interest charges of, 100
scanning laser test billing under, 11–12
use of physician PIN numbers under, 5–6
Medicare -57 modifier, 25

Medicare Carriers Manual, Part 3 Section 2320, 19–20
Medicare/Medicaid services, repaying overpayments for, 97–98, 99–100
Medicare utilization data, to identify coding issues, 59–60

New procedures, overutilization of, 61–62
Off-label use, informed consent for, 69
Office of Inspector General (OIG)
Advisory Opinion No. 00-7 of, 113
compliance documentation guidelines of, 56
compliance guidelines for individual and small group practices of, 67–68
Fraud Alert of, 77–78, 89–90
FY 2002 Work Plan of, 121–122
Model Compliance Program for Individual and Small Group Physician Practices of, 115–116
Office visits, on day of surgery, 25
Ophthalmologist, comanagement contracts of with optometrist, 73–74
Ophthalmoscopy, extended, improper billing for, 37–38
Optical dispensary, Medicare billing issues for, 33–34
Optical services, billing issues for, 33–34
Optometrist
comanagement contracts of with ophthalmologist, 73–74
leasing space from, 77–78
postoperative services of, 75–76
Optometrist-controlled refractive center, 81–82
Overpayments
failure to return, 98
refunding of, 99–100
returning, 97–98
Overutilization, of punctal occlusion with plugs, 61–62

Panretinal photocoagulation, miscoding of, 27–28
Patient counseling, billing for, 29–30
Patient education, about fee arrangements, 79–80
Patient Inducement Prohibition, 112–113, 116
Patient transportation, appropriate use of, 111–113
Patients
new, for physician or practice, 3
return of overpayments by, 98
Payment denial, advance beneficiary notice of, 103–104
Personal identification number (PIN), for billing, 5
Pharmaceutical company relationships, 121–123
inappropriate, 122–123
principles guiding, 122
Physical examinations, documentation score in, 48
Physician Anti-Self-Referral Law. See Stark Law
Physician subcontractors, billing for services of, 91–92
Physician supervision, for diagnostic tests, 107–109
Physicians
joint ventures of, 87–90
responsibility of for obtaining informed consent, 66
responsibility of for patient billing, 67–68
Postcataract surgery glasses, billing for, 33–34
Postoperative YAG capsulotomies, coverage of, 57–58